T0318170

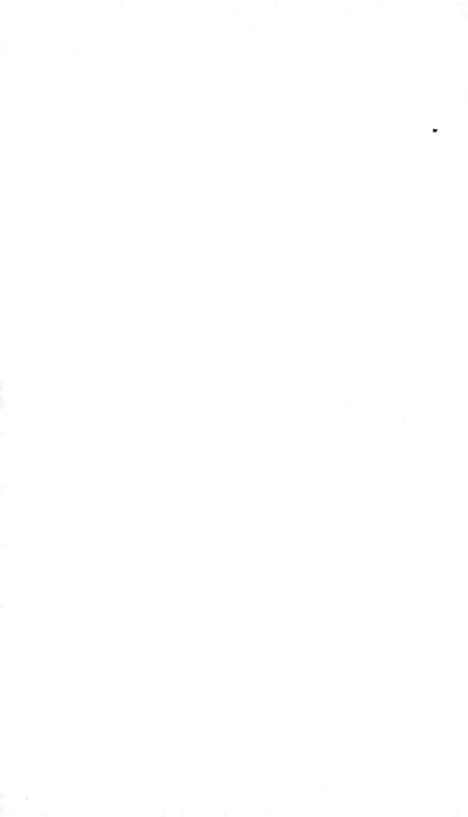

Reaching for Fulfilment as a Woman in Science

This vivid memoir presents adventures from the life of Barbara A. Wilson, an internationally honoured scientist who played an influential role in the development of neuropsychological rehabilitation at a time when the scientific field was dominated by men.

As a follow-up to the highly successful *Story of a Clinical Neuropsychologist*, this book includes a host of memories, both personal and professional, which focus on Barbara's development of her career as a woman in science. From childhood recollections and travels in Africa, to lifetime achievement awards and the restrictions of global pandemics, Barbara tells the story of her full and varied life and her unparalleled career in neuropsychological rehabilitation. Her book indicates that one can lead a meaningful and full life even after one of the most awful of losses, the death of a child, and also emphasizes the need to stick to one's principles in trying times.

The result is an unparalleled insight into the life of a clinical neuropsychologist, which can encourage the next generation of professionals who are trying to balance career, international travel and family, as well as inspire any girls interested in entering the world of science.

Barbara A. Wilson has worked in brain injury rehabilitation for over 42 years. She founded the Oliver Zangwill Centre and the journal *Neuropsychological Rehabilitation*. She has won many awards including an OBE for services to rehabilitation. She is a Fellow of The British Psychological Society, The Academy of Medical Sciences and The Academy of Social Sciences, and honorary professor at the University of Hong Kong, the University of Sydney and the University of East Anglia.

Reaching for Fulfilment as a Woman in Science

Further Stories of a Clinical Neuropsychologist

Barbara A. Wilson

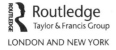

Routledge
Taylor & Francis Group

LONDON AND NEW YORK

First published 2021
by Routledge
2 Park Square, Milton Park, Abingdon, Oxon OX14 4RN

and by Routledge
605 Third Avenue, New York, NY 10017

Routledge is an imprint of the Taylor & Francis Group, an informa business

British Library Cataloguing-in-Publication Data
A catalogue record for this book is available from the British Library

Library of Congress Cataloging-in-Publication Data
A catalog record has been requested for this book

ISBN 13: 978-0-367-56956-3 (pbk)
ISBN 13: 978-0-367-56957-0 (hbk)

Typeset in Times New Roman
by Taylor & Francis Books

Contents

Figures

Acknowledgements

First and foremost, I would like to thank my husband, Mick, for his interest in this book and his willingness to read and comment on everything I send to him. Second, I wish to express my gratitude to Jessica Fish for her constant help and support. I am also very appreciative of the patients who have taught me so much, in particular Kate and Tracey. I also thank Fionnuala Murphy for sending details of the women in science day she organised in Cambridge. Thanks, too, to Routledge for permission to reproduce the story about Tracey in Chapter 14, the editorial in Chapter 20 and the book review in Chapter 18. I am grateful to Philippa Davies, communications manager from Cambridge Community Services NHS Trust, who has given permission to reproduce the piece in their newsletter about me winning the Midland and East award. The World Federation of NeuroRehabilitation kindly allowed me to reproduce the article from their newsletter in Chapter 19. A huge thank you is due to all my friends and colleagues around the world for their willingness to let me reproduce their emails and stories. These include Simon Shorvon for his information on women neurologists; Elkhonon Goldberg for his stimulating webinar on Covid-19, and his story of managing to leave the old Soviet Union; Robyn Tate for her explanations of NeuroBite and the SCRIBE papers; Leigh Schrieff for reminding me of things I had forgotten in South Africa; Juan Carlos Arango for jogging my memory about the workshop in Bogota; my helpful colleague in Argentina, Andrea Querejeta, my lovely Brazilian friends, especially Anita Taub, Fabricia Loschiavo and Eliane Miotto for their collaboration; and similarly from my dear friends from India, Jwala Narayanan, Urvashi Shah, Aparna Dutt, Nithya Hariya-Mohan and Farzana Mulla. Mick and I would also like to thank Helena Chadwick for permission to cite her piece about Venice Manley in Chapter 7. In addition to Jessica and Robyn, my other much-loved friends who have helped me keep sane in this pandemic are Jill Winegardner, Jonathan Evans, Shai Betteridge and Michael Perdices. I thank every one of you. Many thanks to my son, Matt, the photographer for permission to use some of his photographs. Finally, I offer my sincere gratitude to Lucy Kennedy from Routledge for her encouragement in writing this, and her willingness to help throughout the process.

The three poems by Monkwick pupils first appeared in the school's magazine in 1966 edited by Mick. Kay's poem was commended in the BBC's radio programme "Books, Plays, Poems" for its power and skill.

Preface by Mick Wilson

1940 to 2020 – 'The start and finish of an era'

When this autobiography was thought of, and during the writing of its first half, the author, Barbara Wilson, was not thinking about the worldly magnitude of the period of years of her lifetime that can now justifiably be summarised as an *era*; that is a division of time in which 'everything in the world has changed significantly' (*Oxford Dictionary*). The Second World War started a year earlier than 1940 and the world itself was threatened by the pandemic in 2020. As we all know, a lot has happened in between, including a growth in our understanding of the effects of brain injury, to which the author pays attention in this book and for which she is regarded as one of the world's leading experts.

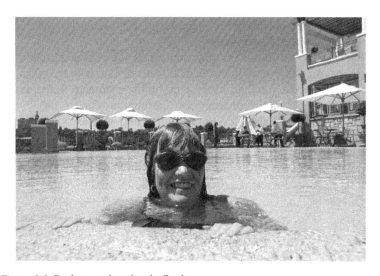

Figure 0.1 Barbara swimming in Spain

Endowed with a remarkable memory herself, dating back to the early 1940s, supported by an extensive daily diary stretching over a period of over four decades, and accompanied by a husband who has always been there for 58 years and still counting, Barbara Wilson has written a second part to her autobiography of a clinical neuropsychologist. It contains memories of a wartime childhood, an education, a profession, an academic discipline, scientific research, travels in all seven continents, a marriage and motherhood; political battles, career success and tragic family loss. It also records ordinary family life during decades in which Britain has attempted to move towards a more civilised society: one in which eventually the death penalty is abolished, homosexuality is decriminalised, suicide regarded as non-criminal; abortion legalised within certain limitations; and greater racial harmony pursued.

As we know from Book One, Barbara's story frequently goes beyond national boundaries as a result of her travels in connection with her professional work as a lecturer, workshop leader and conference speaker. She also travels far afield when holidaying, which includes safaris and beach and island hotel breaks when her ardent if not particularly elegant swimming comes to the fore! To illustrate this point, Barbara learned to swim seriously because she wanted to swim with sea-lions and other creatures that inhabit the Galapagos Islands. Since succeeding in that ambition she has made great use of beautifully decorative hotel pools whenever she can, usually doing a kilometre in her unique and very slow freestyle, frequently observed by other holiday makers with a certain disbelief which turns to amazement when after 40 minutes she is still swimming.

This is, then, an autobiography that offers the reader a story that weaves round the world in its telling. The reader will be taken to another home and into the lives of its family members, learn about neuropsychological rehabilitation for various insults to the brain, causes of and treatments for brain injury; and will learn about the world of scientific research and its application to survivors of brain injury. The reader can travel round the world, visiting some of its treatment centres, its academic meetings, its holiday resorts, and some of its more rugged terrains as well the occasional swish hotel.

Introduction

I am beginning this second book about my memoirs while existing in the middle of the coronavirus pandemic. As I started writing, the lockdown was announced just over four weeks ago, and it is more than five weeks since I stopped going to the gym as we were told then that anyone over the age of 70 years was considered especially vulnerable! At the age of 78, I am one of the fittest and healthiest people I know so I wasn't too pleased that all 70-year-olds were lumped together. Instead of the gym, I go for a 6-mile walk each day and will say more about that later in the book. My husband Mick and I remain healthy in these troubled times as do all our family, although I worry about the effects of this isolation on my 4-year-old great-granddaughter, Amélie, who should be playing with friends, going to nursery and being with her extended family. My surviving daughter, Anna, who is Amélie's grandmother, used to have Amélie for a sleepover every Monday. Recently, Amélie said to Anna 'Will Mondays ever come again?' Anna spends one hour a day on Skype with Amélie but it is not the same as seeing her face to face.

Some of us wonder if we have already had the virus before it was recognised as a problem here in the United Kingdom. Anna was unwell in late January and Mick and I felt ill in February. We didn't have a fever, one of the main symptoms of Covid-19, but we all had a symptomatic cough. Mick's cough was more severe than mine. We said to each other that it was not like a normal cold as we were not sneezing and our noses were not running. We both recovered. Then just as the pandemic was taking off, Mike, Anna's husband was working in London, the worst affected place in the UK. He became ill with all the symptoms of Covid-19 so had to self-isolate, as did Anna. They slept in the same bed but Anna did not become ill so either Mike did not have the coronavirus or else Anna was immune from being ill before. We will never know I guess as none of us has been tested and, at the time of writing, there is no reliable antibody test available. If it does appear we will not be top priority for being tested.

This book is a follow-up to my biography published in 2020. It includes memories, both personal and professional, omitted from the earlier version, and stresses more the fact that I have succeeded in science in what used to be considered a male-dominated world. This was particularly true in the earlier part of my career.

Despite a disadvantaged childhood, I was not unhappy once I returned from an evacuation home in 1944. I write about concerts I arranged in our back garden during those years immediately after the war, adventures with my cousins Peter and June and my learning disabled mother's faux pas. Personal stories as an adult include travel to different continents not previously reported, Mick's arrest in the USA, the Brexit fight, the influence and restrictions of the coronavirus and other stories from both work and play. The bulk of the book, however, focuses on professional work including workshops and conventions in the USA, Japan, Australia, India and South America. I consider the ups and downs of my professional life and reflect on why I have been successful especially in a world where men find success easier than women. In all of this I shall discuss my changing relationships with our children and their children and partners; and my marriage to Mick, including further escapades we had together in various hotels, territories (including jungle, desert, mountains etc.) beaches and swimming pools.

1 Further childhood memories

After I returned from the evacuation home, we lived in Brixton at my grandmother's rented house. She had the downstairs flat and we had the middle floor. I played in the street with the Ransdale children who lived next door and spent a great deal of time dancing. I made up dances that I thought were beautiful. This is ironic as I never dance now, I think I am a rubbish dancer and hate the thought of making a fool of myself, but then I danced and I think it was a way of expressing myself.

At that time, working horses were still used by milkmen and coalmen. Every week, the coalman would come down our street with his coal van and his beautiful carthorse. I used to go out to feed this horse with an apple or a carrot. I loved the horse. I have always been an animal lover and remain so to the present day. Many of the dogs I see on my walks think they know me and come up wagging their tails to be petted or just to be friendly.

Our next move was to Lewis Trust buildings in Camberwell opposite the bus garage which became a playground although we had to be careful not to be caught by the workers there. This was a good place to be an adventurous child even though it was considered to be a very rough area by older people. We really did keep coal in the bath! Our table was actually over the bath which we never used as this is where we kept the coal. Soon after we moved and I was playing in the squares around the flats, I watched a gang of children on the sheds. I wanted to join the gang and play with them but the rule was one could only join once you could climb onto the sheds without help. I was so keen to join I tried really hard and was soon able to pull myself up to the top of the sheds. This was a very proud moment for me.

I know my father had a soft spot for Vera Lynn, the forces' sweetheart as she kept the spirits of the soldiers up during the war. (Vera Lynn died at the age of 103 years on 18 June 2020. Her funeral was held on 10 July.) I didn't realise how much she meant to them until I started jeering at her singing one day when she was on the radio. My father defended her and scolded me so I never jeered at her again. She is still alive at the time of writing in 2020 and is now 103 years old. Each time I see her I think of my dad. He also explained to me about radar and how important this was during the war and how it was discovered after studying bats and their echo location system. My mother was also affected by the war, not just because my father was away for six years, fighting, but because her brother, Ted, was killed in action; I don't think I realised then how upset the family were about this.

When we moved to Foreign Street at Loughborough Junction, I organised concerts in the back garden with my cousin Juney who lived upstairs. I charged friends and relatives to come. I think they paid a penny or two (in old money). I did most of the performances, singing songs and dancing. Juney was not allowed to do much more than collect the money. My favourite song at that time was called 'Down by the Rhine' and it started 'Twas down by the Rhine, I met Caroline. Her hair was so fair and her eyes a shine'. I cannot find this song now on Google so I have no idea where it came from. Another irony is that I thought I could sing! Now, I am known by my family for not being able to sing in tune, although I learn words to songs easily. My musical husband and children either laugh at me or groan when I try to sing. A family joke when the kids were teenagers was for one of them to say 'Mum, go Aah' (and sing a note). I would copy what I thought was the note and they would all laugh. I realised by the time I went to grammar school that I was not singing in tune and thereafter would mouth the words instead of singing out loud. In most circumstances I still do this today.

One day when I was at Crawford Rd primary school and coming home with Juney who was a year younger than me, we decided to eat some privet leaves just to see what they were like and what would happen. They tasted awful of course but the next day we both developed chickenpox which I thought was caused by the privet and for a long time afterwards I told people that eating privet caused chickenpox. It was several years before I realised eating privet and developing chickenpox was simply a coincidence.

Another misadventure occurred on the way home from primary school when I was about 8 years old. A group of us were climbing a fence topped with barbed wire. I slipped and my left hand was trapped on the barbed wire. I screamed and somehow managed to free my hand and get down from the fence. I clasped my right hand over the wound and rushed home to Aunt Vi who was looking after me until my mother returned from work. I would not take my right hand from the wound so Vi had to take me to Kings College Hospital where I was treated. I still have a scar where the barbed wire went in. Later when my father realised I had difficulty telling my left from my right, he asked if I had a scar I could use. To this day I use the scar on my left hand to tell my left from my right. If I am wearing gloves, I imagine the hand with the scar.

I seemed to be attending King's College Hospital regularly. I was once running along a low brick wall and fell off scraping my shin. I looked down and could see white bone in my shin. This was terrifying to me and I was on my own. Then a passing stranger suggested I go to the nearby hospital, King's College. I went and was seen to by a friendly nurse. I told her I really lived on a farm in Scotland and had a beautiful white horse. She pretended to believe me. I was always living in a fantasy world at this time.

Another time, I decided to organise a jumble sale in our house and I made a list of things with their prices to show to anyone who came round. Some workmen came so I decided to show them the list. On it I had listed a butterfly ornament for three pence (less than sixpence in decimal money). One of the workmen asked to see it and bought it. When my father came home from work I told him and he was shocked as I had sold a beautiful ornament for a fraction of its real worth.

I remember my dad teaching me rhyming slang, used by Londoners more then but to some extent the remnants of it are used today. 'Rosie Lee' stands for tea; 'apples and pears' for stairs, 'plates of meat' for feet and 'Bristol City' for titty. Usually the second word in the phrase is omitted so 'I want a cup of Rosie' is used for a cup of tea. I was fascinated by this rhyming slang. My dad also told me about Pearly Kings and Queens as we sometimes saw these at special events. The Kings and Queens, dressed in black with pearl buttons sewn all over their clothes, looked wonderful to me. Originating in the nineteenth century, Pearly Kings and Queens evolved from the Costermonger Kings and Queens, who were elected as leaders of London's street traders (a costard is an apple and a monger a seller). Wikipedia (downloaded 25 April 2020) says 'Costers admired style and panache and with the typical Coster cheek they imitated the wealthy West End society, who by the early nineteenth century had developed a fashion for wearing pearls and parading in their finery on Sundays in the fashionable London parks.' The Costers took it one step further by sewing lines of pearl flashers on their battered hand-me down waist coats, caps and working trousers and started doing their own parade – the 'Lambeth Walk'. I knew the song, 'Lambeth Walk', of course as I lived in Brixton, part of Lambeth. It starts 'Any time you're Lambeth way, any evening, any day, you'll find us all, doing the Lambeth walk'. Later at grammar school, my best friend, Mary Lambert, lived in Walworth and, that too, had its own song 'We are the Walworth girls' I knew all the songs and would belt them out before I realised I could not sing in tune.

While we were still living in Lewis Trust buildings, someone in the royal family came visiting in a special car. All the children lined the streets to wave as the car drove past. Even though my father was anti royalist as I explained in the earlier book, I was allowed to join the others to cheer and wave. Before the parade, we saw from our window in the flats, a man in the square selling wooden rattles for us to buy and twirl when we saw the royal person (I have forgotten just who it was). I wanted one of these rattles so my mother said to go and ask the man how much they were. I went down and asked the man who said they were a tanner. I had no idea that a tanner was a slang word for sixpence so I went upstairs and told my mother the rattles were a tanner. She slapped me for using a slang word! I was allowed to buy one though. We seemed to be a mixture of very rough with aspirations to better ourselves.

As I said in the first book, I loved going to Brownies until I had a row with Brown Owl and left. This reminds me of one of my learning disabled mother's mistakes. At Christmas time she wrote cards to various people and wrote one to 'Brown Ale' instead of 'Brown Owl'. I did not realise she had done this until it was too late so you can imagine how embarrassing that was for me! Another came when she wrote a card to the headmistress of Crawford Road school. Her name was Miss Livesey but behind her back we called her 'Old Liverguts'. Of course my mother wrote the card to Miss Liverguts!

My mother continued to embarrass me when I went to grammar school. She spent almost every Sunday in bed with serious headaches. Only later did I realise she was almost certainly suffering from a hangover on Sundays as she and my father used to go to the Ivy League Club on Saturdays where she drank several gin and tonics. Sometimes I would be left alone and sometimes I would be dragged along with them. I hated the place as it was full of smoke which hurt my eyes; it was also loud and noisy with singing and dancing. I became too tired to walk home so would ride on my dad's shoulders. Once he fell in a hole in the pavement with me on his shoulders. I was fine but my father, no doubt rather drunk, sustained a nasty wound on his hand.

A further embarrassment from my mother occurred when I was a little older perhaps about 10 or 11 years. She regularly sent me to the chemist to purchase some special tablets. For a couple of months or so, I went once a week to get these tablets until one day, the boss man or pharmacist or, at least someone in charge, came to question me. He wanted to know who the tablets were for, did I take any myself and so on. The man told me I would not be allowed to buy any more of these pills. I suspect my mother was taking some addictive substance. I never found out just what but I was not sent again to purchase them. The worst thing I can remember my mother doing was shoplifting! I was a teenager then, about 15 years old and doing a Saturday job, working in a sweetshop. My mother came in very shocked to tell me there had been an incident; she was minding some shopping bags for a woman who hadn't paid and the security man came and she was charged. She had obviously not paid for the shopping and was trying to pretend it was an accident. She was charged and fined and the story appeared in the local newspaper, the *South London Press*. I thought my school friends would learn about my mother and jeer and sneer at me but, as far as I can remember, nobody said a word. My poor mother, a sweet kind rather dumb woman who thought she could get away with stealing. There were obviously semi-criminals on both sides. My mother's cousin or some distant relative called Uncle Speedy, dealt in stolen goods. I can remember him asking my father to keep some stolen suits for him. My father was petrified and went white every time there was a knock on the door. Eventually, Speedy removed the suits and my father would not help him out ever again. I remember Speedy was good at playing spoons. These are knocked one against the other as a poor man's percussion instrument.

My father avoided the police as much as possible. He was born William David Marsh but changed his name as a young man to Forester (my maiden name) when he was possibly running away from the police. He saw a poster of a boxer called Bob Forester (or maybe Forrester as this surname usually has two 'r's in it) and chose this as his new name. My dad's story was pieced together many years later and I now have a copy of the newspaper report about the problem. My father was on a bus and jumped off just before the stop as the bus was slowing down. Many of us have done this including me. However, as my father jumped off the bus, a motor cyclist with a young woman riding pillion, came along. The motor bike swerved to avoid my father, the young woman was thrown off and was killed. My father was not charged as he had not committed a crime but he was seen before magistrates and cautioned. This, you might think, is no reason to change your name but it is possible that the young woman's family or the motor cyclist were seeking revenge. Whatever the reason, Bill changed his name to Forester, never obtained a passport and kept out of trouble as far as he could. My mother was horrified when she learned later of the name change thinking they were not legally married. She checked this out and learned that their marriage was indeed legal. So was my maiden name. My father went through the war as William David Forester and fought in France and Germany (presumably one did not need passports when fighting abroad with the army). He died as a Forester and not a Marsh although this name change caused me a headache when I was trying to obtain my Irish citizenship many years later. I return to this story in a later chapter.

The final piece of shady behaviour I remember from my schooldays was to do with my Irish grandmother's second 'husband' known as 'Old Wonk Eye' as he lost an eye in the First World War. This man was not my real grandfather but that is what I called him. I would see him on the Brixton Road sometimes and say 'Hello granddad' to which he always replied 'Who's are you?' I would reply, 'I am Bill's'. This seemed normal to me at the time as it always happened. Anyway, the story was that if someone we knew was charged by the police, they could go to see Old Wonk Eye who would sort it out at Brixton Police Station. Rumour had it that a bribe would be paid and the charge dropped. How true this really was, I do not know, but it was firmly believed by my father and others that Old Wonk Eye and the police had a special arrangement.

It was while at grammar school that I learned to speak more correctly. One of the teachers told us that we would not get on in life if we did not modify our speech so I started to change my accent, at least while I was at school. In fact, I had two accents, one for school and one for home. Now I only ever revert to the very rough one when I am very angry or for a joke.

From the age of about 13 years, I usually rode to school on a bicycle. I enjoyed these cycle rides and my parents had bought me a bicycle on hire purchase for a Christmas present. I was allowed to choose the bike I wanted from a cycle shop and chose one with straight handlebars that was kingfisher blue in colour. I loved this bike and proudly went to pay the weekly money for the hire purchase agreement. I was also proud of it when I went to school. It was a very treasured possession. One day, visiting my grandmother's house in Brixton, I left the bike outside. Later when I went to collect it, it wasn't there. I was panic stricken and thought the bike had been stolen. I was about to go inside and tell my mother when I saw my aunt Bet, one of my mother's sisters, riding the bike at the end of the street! She just wanted to try it out. It was a great relief that my treasured bike had not been stolen.

One final story from grammar school days is about a mantra told us by the headmistress, Miss Hay, a Scottish and very religious person. She came to the school when I was in the third form, I believe. Before that we had Miss Shaw, a very obese person. Miss Hay would frequently say to us: 'Girls, remember your body is a temple for the holy ghost. (pause) What is your body?' We duly chanted back, 'A temple for the holy ghost, Miss.' Of course, we had no idea what this meant. It seemed like a joke. Later, I realised she probably meant we weren't allowed to have sex but this was never spelled out.

2 Early marriage

I have written at length in the first book about going to Teacher Training College and meeting up with Mick, marrying him while we were both working at the Royal School for Deaf Children in Margate, our first year of marriage, and the birth of Sarah in Ramsgate Hospital. There are a few more things I'd like to write about those days. After a brief separation, Mick and I started going out together again in 1961 and I started work as a housemother at The Royal School for Deaf Children in Margate. We had to keep our relationship secret from the members of staff at the school as Mick was a teacher and it was looked down upon for teachers to fraternise with housemothers. Our courting was done at Dreamland, the Margate amusement park, where we listened to Acker Bilk's Jazz Band among others and I remember being very cold as we walked back to our separate accommodations at the school. There was one pub we frequented and initially, always requested our song to be played by the pianist. The song was 'Smoke gets in your eyes'. We were soon recognised and this song played as we walked in the door.

Mick and I married in July 1962, hitchhiked to Cornwall for our honeymoon where I fell off the cliffs and spent three nights in Truro hospital and had our first baby, Sarah, ten and a half months later. At that time, to set our story in an historical context, the UK still had capital punishment and homosexuality was illegal. The last woman to be hanged was Ruth Ellis in 1955. I was at school then and remember being shocked. We all hoped she would be pardoned and there was a public petition supporting this but she was hanged. I believe that the awfulness of capital punishment was then realised more fully by society and moves in Parliament were started to end this barbaric practice. The hanging of the last two men, Peter Anthony Allen and Gwynne Owen Evans was in August 1964. This was after our marriage, after the birth of Sarah and a month before Anna was born. Other men were condemned to death but their sentences commuted to life imprisonment. This capital punishment for murder was still in fact legal until 1969 and allowed as a punishment for treason until 1998!

Many years later, in 2006, I was in Texas receiving the Robert Moody award for contributions to brain injury rehabilitation. Moody, a wealthy man, had a son who had sustained a traumatic brain injury and thereafter funded treatment and research into traumatic brain injury rehabilitation. I was the first non-American to receive this award and was invited to give an address and receive the award at a conference. After the meeting, I went to a dinner hosted for the conference attendees. During the conversation at dinner, the issue of the death penalty came up. Remember this was in America with a much higher murder rate than the UK and an equally high rate of capital punishment, with Texas being the state with the most number of executions carried out for those who had committed or were thought to have committed homicides. At the dinner, some Americans were saying it was good to have the death penalty as it acted as a deterrent. One well known psychologist said it certainly deterred him. I thought, and should have said, that I did not need a deterrent to stop me killing someone!

Another milestone that occurred in the early years of our marriage was the decriminalisation of homosexuality. This occurred in 1967 after the Wolfenden Report which was published in 1957. Mick told me that some years earlier Wolfenden himself came to Mick's all boys grammar school, in the early 1950s, to talk about the need to end criminalisation of homosexuality. In fact, Mick remembers that this subject had never been raised by teachers in all the six years previously: it seems to have been a forbidden topic in an all boys' school in those days. Mick reflects that, at most, there must have been two or three recognised homosexual boys at the school when in fact of course there would have been many more, but as it was criminalised, each would be petrified to mention the fact. He remembers Wolfenden being a very impressive speaker, although homosexuality never became a subject for discussion amongst the sixth formers in the early 1950s. Legalisation had to come!

One of the saddest stories was that of the brilliant Alan Turing, a Cambridge mathematician and computer scientist who helped us win the Second World War through breaking a major code used by the Germans to such an impressive extent that battles were lost by us before the code was broken. Turing was prosecuted for homosexuality in 1952. He accepted chemical castration instead of going to prison and died just before his 42nd birthday in 1954 through cyanide poisoning. This was thought to be a suicide attempt but could have been accidental poisoning. Wikipedia (downloaded 3 May 2020) report that: 'in 2009, following an Internet campaign, British prime minister Gordon Brown made an official public apology on behalf of the British government for the appalling way Turing was treated'. Queen Elizabeth II granted Turing a posthumous pardon in 2013. The "Alan Turing law" is now an informal term for a 2017 law in the United Kingdom that retroactively pardoned men cautioned or convicted under historical legislation that outlawed homosexual acts'. The prime minister who was in power when homosexuality was legalised in 1967 was Harold Wilson. He remained prime minister until 1970 by which time both our daughters were at school. Having the same surname, they claimed he was their grandfather and had several of their friends believing this!

With three young children and always short of money, we frequently holidayed with Mick's Suffolk friends, Mike and Sue Crooks. They had a beautiful house and a very large garden where we camped. Mike made his money once he became a very successful auctioneer. Before that Mick and Mike had worked together years before, digging all day with a shovel and pickaxe for hours and hours on end to complete foundations for buildings. There were many labourers employed in this way on each building site, very hard grafting. All of this work is now done by a single machine on each site at great speed. When was the last time anyone saw a shovel on a building site I wonder?

The Crooks had three young children having tragically lost their firstborn son in an accident when he was about a year old. He was crawling across the floor, sucked on an electrical socket and electrocuted himself. I found Mike a bit of a male chauvinist and felt he favoured his two boys over his daughter as I heard him once say to his sons about his daughter, 'she's only a girl'. This was not welcome to me but I kept quiet partly because I am naturally polite and partly because Mick liked Mike because of their long time spent in back-breaking work. I liked Sue, Mike's wife, but thought she did not stand up for herself enough.

Sue owned some property, a small nightclub, in Ipswich and one day a man approached Mike with a view to buying the property to make into a restaurant. Straightaway, Mike became interested and arranged to meet the man's friend but his enthusiasm turned immediately sour when the man said, 'By the way, the would-be purchaser is Charlie, brother to the Kray twins.' (The Kray twins were notorious British criminals.)

Mike's mood changed as they drove the car to Bramford where the brothers lived. However, Mike's chat with the Krays was amicable and business like, although his heart was pounding and he wanted to get out of any deal which might follow. Nothing came of it eventually though as the Ipswich Council would not allow the property to be used as a restaurant and it had to remain a nightclub. The Krays lost interest and a curious explanation Mick was told eventually was that nightclubs could be invaded by the police and restaurants could not.

Makes you think doesn't it? One last parting shot (if you'll excuse the unintended pun) was Charlie's goodbye to Mike which included a goodwill gesture when he said, 'If you ever get into trouble the first one will be on us.'

Mick's progress as Head of English at Monkwick County Secondary school continued and he was frequently consulted and advised by the county inspectorate, in particular by David Caruth who was responsible for overseeing the teaching of English throughout the county of Essex. The system of county inspectors was a good one and helped to improve the quality of education throughout England. It was positive and non-threatening. Aiming to improve the quality of teaching and learning in the classroom, inspectors and teachers were all members of the same team working together, unlike today's system where inspectors are remote from schools except when they do actually inspect them and pronounce judgements through Ofsted. Now, apparently, they can do this without providing notice – which, to Mick, sounds very threatening!

The 1960s was a great decade to be teaching and Mick regards it as a 'golden age'. There was some wonderful work being done in primary schools and the new examination, the Certificate for Secondary Education was stimulating creative and pupil-led learning in secondary classrooms. Problem solving rather than pseudo lecturing was becoming the norm in leading schools of this era. Things changed at an extremely fast pace as many secondary schools were being staffed, ironically, by bright young teachers who had attended grammar schools themselves, gone on to a university education and been influenced by all kinds of educationists and writers such as Richard Hoggart, David Holbrook, Ted Hughes, Harold Rosen, Connie Rosen, Douglas Barnes and James Britton, many of whom influenced the government report 'A Language for Life' which argued for each school having an original policy for language across the curriculum.

At the same time popular culture was changing at an equally fast rate and Mick can remember using the songs of Bob Dylan in certain poetry lessons rather than some of those long ballads about knights in shining armour and maidens in distress! Learning was being based on the lives of pupils and the localities where they lived. So different from the hated regimes that existed in some earlier secondary modern schools where discipline rather than learning was the goal.

To give you an idea of the freedom and creativity that was being encouraged in education in the 1960s here is how marks were obtained at the CSE, designed by Mick, at the end of two year's study:

60 per cent – course work
20 per cent – open book examination lasting all day, pupils were allowed to consult books
20 per cent – oral work based on contributions in the classroom over the two years.

At the same time the GCE offered two three-hour exams after two years studying formal ways of writing and one novel, one play and one book of poems, taking two whole years to study! Mick's pupils had their own reading diaries where they wrote reviews of each book they read privately and out of school. At the same time they would do some class reading of books such as *The Catcher in the Rye, Huckleberry Finn, Lord of the Flies*, and *Of Mice and Men*, and some of the short stories of Doris Lessing.

Mick's pupils kept reading and film viewing diaries, had their own British Film Institute supported film club; acted *Midsummer Night's Dream* at the end of two years as the school play attended by parents, did a class reading of *Macbeth*, and went to Stratford to see *Henry IV Part One*. Mick also produced a dance drama attended by parents, based on *The Tempest*. And this was all in a secondary modern school that, as far as the general public, the mass media, parents and politicians, were concerned, was supposed to be interested only in discipline, woodwork for the boys and domestic science for girls! (Interesting that they called housework a 'science'!)

I'd like to provide a few examples of the pupil's creative writing to give the readers an idea of the quality of some of the pupil's work in Mick's classes, so maybe I'll do that next? But remember if I do that these pupils were considered by some members of society to be failures once they had failed the 11+. I wonder what the brilliant actor Patrick Stewart thinks of that as he was one of those kids? In fact there are many very successful people who went on to contribute in higher education and various other professions despite having failed a test at the age of 11 years.

This is a poem written by Kay Quigley, who was in the third year at the time so she would have been about 13 years old. Remember this was the 1960s and we'd had the Cuba crisis when Russia and the USA almost went to war over Russia's intention to build nuclear bases there – right next door to the USA!

Cold black hideous steel
Clanking throbbing bobs and gadgets
Rending bolts pumping pushing -
Cold black and hideous.

Feed its mouth brassy and hot
Feed its mouth with intelligence
Give it more knowledge, train its brain

Feed its mouth, with life.

See if it can walk,
See if it can walk the floor unaided
Beckon it, call it

See if it can walk to you.

Take it outside
Take it outside and show it the world,
Show it mankind death and hatred
Take it to the world outside.

Teach it death and hatred
Teach it death and watch its gadgets throb,
Why does it cower at us? It's more intelligent?
Quick teach it death and hatred.

Even he cannot learn
Even he cannot learn the art of death
We only know this art alone
Even he cannot learn.

Leave the thing at peace
Leave the thing we have tried to teach.
It had the power to overthrow us all;
Don't teach it all we know.
Cold back and hideous – leave the thing at peace.
                    KAY QUIGLEY 3III

In contrast, here is something else, written this time by 14-year-old Colin. The class was encouraged to write with their FIVE senses as urged by Ted Hughes in one of his BBC broadcasts for children.

I walked home along the cold, dark road. It was a cold night with stars shining occasionally through the clouds. I was cold and hungry. I began to think about what I might have for tea: soup, steaming hot, with sausages and potatoes covered in thick, brown gravy. A nice cup of tea, and to finish up with some hot rice. These thoughts made me hungrier and made me hurry. The thoughts went round and round. My mouth was full of these tastes and it watered so much that I had a job to swallow it. I could see my house now, so faster and faster I went. I reached the back door. I opened it and there on the table was a plate of sandwiches with a note saying, 'I have gone to Miss Smith's funeral, Mum.'

An anonymous poem by R.C. (13?)

I sit for endless hours
Of well told stories.
My dad, my dad, my dad.
First it's Russia then Australia.
Now he's under mortar fire.
I sit there taking words and
sentences in,
Wondering when I may retire.
But it's on and on it never stops.
I wish, if only I could turn him off.
But it's easier said than done.
Television's good but that's no use,
The film's on, 'Lost in the desert'
But my dad, well he's in Iceland
By gad, I've had it.

There is something that I can add to the text here this very minute as we have just received our copy of today's *Guardian* (10 July 2020). Mick grabbed the newspaper eagerly because he had written a letter to them which he hoped would be published today. It is not published and Mick is disappointed. But I think it's applicable to what I've just written so I'll include it here. It's based on the fact that many of the famous actor Patrick Stewart's friends had been interviewed in yesterday's *Guardian* to celebrate his 80th birthday. Mick's letter is as follows:

The interviews with friends of Patrick Stewart were a joy to read (Guardian, 9 July) illuminating his superb acting skills and personality, 'his wryness, wisdom, sensitivity' and his sense of fun. Nobody however mentioned the fact that Patrick was initially educated at a secondary modern school to which he has always shown allegiance. Patrick unfailingly singles out Mr. Dormand (always referred to as 'Sir') who he praises for his 'dedication, warmth and inspirational teaching'. We need reminding that there were some great teachers in some secondary modern schools, as well, of course as some brilliant students.

Signed: Mick Wilson, Bury St Edmunds

3 Women in science

In the earlier book, I talk about going to university as a mature student at the age of 30 when our youngest child, Matthew, had just started school; then my clinical training and how I discovered brain injury rehabilitation when I started work at Rivermead Rehabilitation Centre in Oxford. I knew after my first day there that this is the work I wanted to do for the rest of my career. I also described leading what was probably the only successful occupation of a health service facility. I think this shows that I have never been afraid to fight for what I believe is right. I am ambitious in some ways, but know that I am more interested in improving the lives of brain injured people and their families, than I am in furthering my career. During my clinical training I was told that every patient seen should be capable of being written up for a journal and that no patient is untestable. I was taught the science-practitioner model, that everything we do should be evaluated and was instilled with the value of writing up our work. This was confirmed by my boss in Oxford, John Hall. He said there was no point in doing things if we did not tell the world about it. Consequently, I have always felt the need to write and to at least attempt to evaluate the rehabilitation given to people. I have also been willing to attend international conferences and present my work even if on many occasions I had to pay for myself. Both the writing and the attendance at conferences have paid off and are reasons why I am known and appreciated around the world.

Most undergraduates in psychology are women but most psychologists in senior positions are men. Three incidents stand out in my mind here illustrating the relative rarity of women in senior positions. One is a conference organised by Fionnuala Murphy in Cambridge called 'Women in Science'. It happened because of a quinquennial (5 year) review of the Medical Research Council's Cognition and Brain Sciences Unit in Cambridge. This was after I had formally retired from the unit. At the review one of the people evaluating the past five-year work output of the staff there, was a woman, Susan Gathercole, who was later to become Unit Director, the one and only time a woman has been director. There were no female senior scientists attending the review as there were no female senior scientists then employed at the unit (although there were when I worked there and I was one of them). Susan Gathercole asked where the women were. It is unclear whether the male director, William Marslen-Wilson, understood the significance of the question but some of the more junior female staff, including my honorary 'adopted daughter', Jessica Fish, asked if I would speak at a one-day conference organised by Fionnuala Murphy. This was to be a meeting of former female senior scientists including some prestigious people including Dorothy Bishop, Karalyn Patterson, Bundy Mackintosh, Sophie Scott, Nilli Lavie, Elisabeth Hill and Anne Cutler. I spoke about my journey and achievements including the founding of the Oliver Zangwill Centre for Rehabilitation in Ely and the centre in Quito, Ecuador, named after me.

The second incident was to do with the Academy of Medical Sciences of which I was elected a fellow in 2001. Several years later, this academy organised a meeting in Birmingham called 'Women and the Glass Ceiling'. It was to feature women who had broken through the metaphorical glass ceiling and to say why they had succeeded. I was one of the women who agreed to speak. It was an interesting day and my talk was similar to the one I had given at the Cambridge meeting. At the end of the day, we were asked to give three tips for succeeding in science to the mostly young women in the audience. These are the tips I mention at the end of the previous book. Whereas the others said things like find a good laboratory to work for and publish in high-impact journals, I suggested they should not be afraid to fight the system; secondly, to do what they feel passionate about and, three, find a supportive partner. I reminded the audience that our main purpose in life was not to further our careers but to work for the benefit of people with brain injury and their families.

The third incident is not to do with me but concerns a much admired older colleague and friend, Dr Pauline Monro, a retired neurologist. Pauline was the first woman ever to be appointed a consultant at St George's Hospital in London. It is hard to believe that this did not happen until as late as 1971when she took up the post. Not only was Pauline the first woman consultant at the hospital, she also went on to transform the small neurology department into one of the best regional neurology centres in the country. She had a struggle to do this at a time of financial constraints, and on two occasions had to save the neurology beds from the clutches of the neurosurgeons. When Pauline trained in medicine only 10 per cent of students were women and she was told, on more than one occasion, that as a woman she could not expect ever to be appointed as a consultant neurologist. Pauline said that, although she did not experience discrimination among neurologists, throughout her career she quite frequently encountered attitudes and demeaning remarks which would not have been directed at a man.

In 2000 Pauline was awarded an MBE for her work after retirement from the NHS, in improving neurology care in Russia. In 2002 she was awarded a medal from the Association of British Neurologists for her significant contribution to neurology. Warlow (2002) summarised her career, stating that she was an outstanding medical student, gaining a first class honours degree at University College and then a distinction in medicine and pathology when she qualified in 1958. Warlow also remembers Pauline as a wonderful teacher. She went into neurology after hearing J.Z. Young give the Reith lectures. Pauline was still at school at the time of the lectures. In 1969, at the age of 35 she sustained an almost fatal life-changing assault on her nervous system, which left her with mobility problems that became worse with advancing years.

In 2018, long after Pauline's retirement, there was a move to have the neurology ward at St George's named after her in recognition of her achievements but this failed and she was instead made a fellow of the University of London, St George's. In fact, this was the second attempt to name a ward after her. The first time was on her actual retirement. This failed too. However, in St Petersburg the first stroke unit in Russia staffed by a multidisciplinary team was opened in 1998, and subsequently named after Pauline and her husband. This unit was in Pavlov's St Petersburg First Medical University, where Pauline was awarded an honorary degree. She was given a European woman of achievement award in 2004.

I first met Pauline in, I think, 2006 at a dinner after a talk I gave at the Royal Society of Medicine in London. Pauline came up to me at the dinner, said she had greatly enjoyed my talk, and that the approach to neuropsychological rehabilitation I had described was exactly what the Russian neurologists needed to hear. She asked me if I would be interested in giving a talk in Russia? At that time Pauline had already, for many years, been introducing to Russian medical professionals caring for people with acquired disabling neurological disorders, the principles of evidence based medicine, and patient problem-based multidisciplinary team care. These concepts were new to the Russians, who, while working in a well-developed national health system, were prevented from access to overseas colleagues during the Soviet Union period. Although Pauline had, since 1995, been organising two way training and experience exchanges for all other professions members of the neurology MDT, with translation of relevant texts, neuropsychology and neuropsychological rehabilitation had not been included.

Of course, I said I would accept as I had never been to Russia and, being a serious traveller, I wanted to know what it was like. I went the following year to St Petersburg. I learned that Pauline spoke fluent Russian and, to show how good her Russian was, it was thought by some of the locals that she was a native speaker who had lived abroad a long time. This is a language she learned after her retirement in order to be able to communicate with Russian participants in the exchanges she was organising.

Pauline had first been to Leningrad (later renamed St Petersburg) in 1988 with her husband, Michael (who died in 2000) to attend a joint meeting of the Association of British Neurologists and Soviet neurologists. Both Pauline and her husband had long been fascinated by the country because of its major contribution to European music and literature. At that meeting and on subsequent visits Pauline became aware of the effect on patient care of the lack of use of proven effective care methods. A request from two local neurologists in 1992 for foreign neurological literature, eventually led to Pauline setting up, on behalf of the Association of British Neurologists and with the cooperation of Russian neurologists, the Anglo-Russian neurological partnership, in which the previously mentioned exchanges were organised. These were initially funded mainly by a series of grants from the now sadly defunct, UK Department for International Development Know How Fund.

While on my first trip to Russia, I realised what an impressive person Pauline is. She thinks nothing of engaging in the Russian equivalent of hitchhiking (except one pays the driver a small amount at the end of the journey and can end up with some appalling drivers and cars in bad repair); she knows all about Russian culture including opera and ballet, she fights her corner. Pauline told me how, with the help of St Gregory's charity, discarded curtains, round beds, soap and soap dispensers, were distributed in bedside stroke units in St Petersburg. Warlow (2002) reported that chairs and aids to daily living were transported across Europe and that driving across Europe to St Petersburg in a renovated London Ambulance filled with Zimmer frames was more exciting than holding a neurology out-patient clinic.

One of the really interesting places we visited in St Petersburg was the Beloselsky-Belozersky Palace which, from 1916 until 1918, housed the Anglo-Russian Hospital (ARH) in the city which was then called Petrograd. In 1993, Michael Harmer – whose father was Senior Surgeon leading the British staff in the ARH – hearing of Pauline's frequent trips to Russia – had asked for help in creating a memorial plaque in the BB Palace to recognise the work of the ARH. Pauline, with the help of many Russian colleagues and friends, arranged for a plaque to be made and it was unveiled in 1986 on the wall of the Palace (which had by now become a museum) in the presence of descendants of the ARH staff.

I know my approach to rehabilitation was criticised by some of the local Russians as they felt it was not sufficiently influenced by Luria. Luria was a wonderful neuropsychologist and a friend of Oliver Zangwill after whom I named our rehabilitation centre. In fact, I dedicated my first talk in Russia to Luria who died in 1977. I said at one of my talks that if Luria were here today he would want us to move on. Another criticism I faced was that I treated the person and not the brain! To me this is a compliment rather than a criticism as there is no evidence we can treat the brain but plenty of evidence that we can make lives better for the person and his or her family. I have been to Russia several times since then as part of the two way training exchanges organised by Pauline both in St Petersburg and in Moscow. Both are beautiful cities although St Petersburg is my favourite. I was about to go to Nizhniy Novgorod once but Mick was diagnosed with prostate cancer and starting his treatment at the time I was supposed to leave so I cancelled that trip and have not been back. I have not been to Russia for a few years now partly because it is so problematic obtaining visas and partly because I dislike Putin so much. Until the lockdown with the coronavirus, however, Pauline continued to go back and forth to Russia and fight for the improvement of services.

Rehabilitation in Russia has, I think, improved. Pauline certainly believes it has. I have met some fantastic people including Olga Komaeva, a very special person and Vera Grigoryeva from Nizhniy Novgorod. Both are neurologists with an interest in clinical neuropsychology and have played key roles in introducing improvements in Russian neuropsychological rehabilitation. Vera has an identical twin who is also a neurologist. Pauline says this can be confusing at meetings sometimes. Pauline is a modest person and wrote to me saying that

> in all the exchanges with Russia it is the amazing and inspiring specialists, of whom you are an outstanding example, who have given up their time and energy to go to Russia, and hand on their

experience and skills to colleagues there. It is you, who are so inspiring and deserving of admiration, and maybe, even more, so the truly wonderful Russians like Olga Komaeva, who have 'seen the light', absorbed and passed on new knowledge and skills, overcome resistance and, against all the odds, transformed the approaches to people with acquired disabling disorders of the CNS, and undoubtedly improved patient outcome. (email 13 May 2020)

I have been to superb operas and ballets in Russia as Pauline always treats her overseas speakers to one of these. Russian hospitality is good and I admire many of the people. However, I have also seen some pretty awful things too including some Dickensian hospitals and poor treatment of survivors of brain injury. I have introduced others to Pauline and she has invited them to take part in the training exchanges in Russia. Pauline tells me that in recent years the seminars and teaching of our very dear friends, Jill Winegardner, Jonathan Evans, Jessica Fish and Shai Betteridge, has been pivotal in finally, after 13 years of exchanges in clinical neuropsychology, led to the Russians enthusiastically embracing the approach to neuropsychological rehabilitation as proposed at the Oliver Zangwill Centre.

For the Oliver Zangwill Centre fifteenth-year anniversary, a conference was organised at Hinxton Hall in Cambridgeshire and Pauline arranged to bring a party of Russians over. Her grants from the Anglo-Russian neurological partnership would cover the travel but they had no money for accommodation. The staff at the Oliver Zangwill Centre met to decide who could put up the visitors. At the time we lived in a five-bedroomed house with two additional sofa beds one in each of our two sitting rooms so we decided we could take five people. They arrived each with a bottle of vodka. The first night we had a party at our house with all the other staff and visiting Russians coming in a hired minivan. We had a great time with Russian champagne and vodka plus decent food that the British had organised. Mick and I were dreading the visit because of the crowding and the feeding but we ended up thoroughly enjoying ourselves. The lovely Olga, a neurologist, an occupational therapist and a physiotherapist all rolled into one, who continues to this day in teaching MDT care all over Russia and the former Soviet Union, was allocated one of the sofa beds and I felt a bit bad about this. I said to her that I was sorry she had to sleep on a sofa bed. Olga said that in Russia they had no space and shared things so it was no hardship for her to sleep on the sofa bed.

Mick made porridge every morning and the Russians loved it saying 'Meeck, your porridge is wonderful. It is just like our kasha'. They did not ask if they could help with washing up, they just got on and did it. The conference went well and we had planned to go to Brown's in Cambridge for our final meal at the end of the conference but, by then, we were all so tired, I phoned Mick and said that we could not go to Cambridge so he would have to cook for us instead. He went out and bought fish and chips for everyone. We had some of the Russian champagne left from the party so we had that with our fish and chips. It turned out to be a great meal and we had really enjoyed our Russian visitors, who felt honoured at eating real fish and chips!

The point of this long section on Pauline and the Russians is that if I think I have had to struggle being a woman in a man's world, others like Pauline, have had it worse and triumphed.

I was writing this section while reading the scholarly, detailed and fascinating history of the National Hospital, Queen Square (Shorvon & Compston 2019). I decided to email Simon Shorvon to see if the first female consultancy at that hospital occurred before or after Pauline's appointment. Simon, another friend of Pauline's, replied almost immediately saying that 'the first female consultants in Queen Square were two anaesthetists Olive Jones and Edith Margaret Taylor appointed in 1935, so long before Pauline's appointment. Another notable woman was Dr Marjorie Blandy, the first woman registrar at the National Hospital. She was the subject of an excellent book called "Breaking Bounds: six Newnham women" (Tomalin et al. 2014)'. This book gives some details of Dr Blandy's amazing WWI work. It is interesting that female registrars were only allowed at Queen Square first in WWI due to the dearth of available males.

In fact Dr Blandy trained at the London School of Medicine for women in 1909. This was the first medical school in England where women could train (Lefanu 2014) The first outstanding female neurologist in Britain was probably Honor Smith, who moved with Hugh Cairns to Oxford, during WWII. She was a fascinating figure who used to do ward rounds it is said in her hunting gear. Pauline Monro may have been the second female neurologist – who was also a great friend of mine – and, as you know, was indefatigable in promoting British–Russian neurological contacts – and one of the last times I saw her was when by chance I bumped into her at the Opera in St Petersburg.

Simon Shorvon's account was much appreciated and I really like the book he wrote with Alistair Compston but it is notable how few women have been consultants at the National Hospital. One exception is Elizabeth Warrington who was appointed in 1953 and made a professor of clinical neuropsychology in 1982. Elizabeth has contributed greatly to neuropsychology and is admired throughout the world for her insights and theoretical contributions to the field. Simon Shorvon went on to add in his email that people from the black and Asian ethnic minority were appointed many years before any women were appointed as doctors (the first were Brown-Sequard in 1859 and Risien Russell in 1898) and Jewish doctors (the first was John Zachariah Laurence in 1860).These are all described in the Shorvon and Compston book (2019).

Thus, there is a whole history of women in science literature which makes my journey seem tame as I never really experienced overt sexism in my career. I went to an all-girl's school which never taught us to consider ourselves as second-class citizens but I will return to this theme later in the book. Perhaps, the place where I was made most aware of the supposed 'inferior' status of women was in a Mormon household in Salt Lake City, Utah. Utah is a very beautiful state and Mick and I have had wonderful trips in Zion National Park and Bryce Canyon in Southern Utah but I was in Salt Lake City to give a lecture at Brigham Young University. Before the lecture we had to have prayers said (and remember I am a non-believer) but I politely stood while being prayed over. I stayed with a Mormon family, the family of the man who had invited me. I knew that alcohol was forbidden and that was not a big hardship but I had not known that coffee was also off limits! That was difficult for me. When the wife of the household was preparing the evening meal, I asked if I could help and I was given vegetables to chop. I had not really expected to do this as I was, after all, a visiting lecturer. The roles were firmly divided though between the men and the women. I suppose what shocked me the most was a discussion about female education, I was told that the girls were allowed to go to university to do an undergraduate degree but strongly discouraged from doing a higher degree. The boys, however were allowed to do this! Again, I was polite but vowed never to stay with a Mormon family again.

4 My first job as a qualified clinical psychologist

Before I became involved in brain injury rehabilitation, I worked in developmental learning disability or, as it was called then, mental handicap. Recently, while looking through my journals to help me remember things for this book, I found a piece I wrote about a typical day at Hilda Lewis House (HLH), Bethlem Royal Hospital where I worked for three days a week after qualifying; the other two days I worked at the Institute of Psychiatry (IoP) teaching neuropsychology. I had completely forgotten I had ever written this and thought it might be interesting for readers to learn what a typical day was like at HLH for a clinical psychologist in 1977 so I'm including it here. HLH was a special unit for children with severe behaviour problems and often self-injurious behaviour. At the time we were living in Reading, Berkshire.

> The alarm goes at six a.m and I force myself out of bed about ten past six. I never get used to getting up so early and envy my husband and children fast asleep in their warm beds *(It seems odd to say that now in 2020 as I typically wake before 5.15 a.m!)*. I listen to 'farming today' as I get dressed and make my cup of coffee. It is not that I am interested in farming but I use it to pace myself and when 'Today' starts at 6.30 a.m I know that I must start making drinks for the others. At 6.40 a.m, I do my rounds: tea for my husband Mick and my 14 year old daughter, Anna; coffee for my older daughter Sarah who is 15; and orange juice for my son, Matthew who is 12. At 6.45 I set off for the railway station, usually walking two stops down the road before catching the bus in order to save two pence! The journey to work is so expensive, I try to save the odd few pence here and there. At Reading station, I catch the 7.17 train, which stops at Twyford, Maidenhead and Paddington. It reaches Paddington about 8.00 a.m if it is on time. I sometimes catch a bus to Camberwell and sometimes take the underground to

the Elephant and Castle and then another bus from there to Camberwell. I am boycotting the underground as far as possible as it is so expensive but sometimes the buses are so full at Paddington that I am in danger of missing the hospital coach from the Maudsley Hospital (which is next door to the IoP) to Bethlem, the last stage of the journey. I usually reach the Maudsley about 8.50 and may have breakfast there, if time. The hospital coach leaves at 9.05 a.m and reaches Bethlem at 9.35. I then have to walk to the other side of the hospital grounds before finally reaching work at 9.45 a.m. This is three hours after leaving home! (so, with a three hour journey back home at the end of the day and seven hours actually working on the job, I'm putting in a 13 hour day. Then I also work on the journey, either writing one or two reports on a home or school visit or an assessment. I also read references for the next tutorial I am giving at the IoP. On the two IoP days, I leave home with my children at 7.45 a.m and reach the IoP at 10.00 a.m.

Once at work at Bethlem, I rush from one thing to another frantically trying to accomplish everything I need to do before the hospital coach leaves for the Maudsley at 5.10 p.m. I really ought to be sylph like with all the rushing around I do. Although I am not sylph like I am not overweight even though I do eat three cooked meals a day.

I will now describe a typical day, a Tuesday, at Bethlem Royal Hospital. First thing I do after arriving is collect the post. Then I might telephone a teacher about a boy who has left the unit recently and is causing problems at school. This is followed by a case conference to discuss a child I have assessed and been working with. We then plan a treatment programme for the child discussed at the case conference. I run this meeting (a psychologist always runs the treatment programme meetings). After discussion with other members of the team, we decide what the main problems are, how we are going to tackle each problem and who is going to do what. I write this up and take it to the secretaries to type up and distribute to all members of the team *(remember this was in the days before personal computers and we wrote things by hand to be given in for typing)*.

All the children are looked after in small groups with each group having its own psychologist. So, before lunch I go to see the children I am responsible for and check on one boy in particular to see how he is getting on with his ability to feed himself. Next task is to go to the canteen to buy and eat my own lunch before dashing back for the group meeting at 1.00 p.m. At the group meeting, we discuss each child's progress and whether any changes need to be made to the treatment programme. Immediately after the meeting, I write a summary of the changes in the communication book. We have a psychology student on placement so I go to observe her with one of the children before meeting the parents of a girl on the unit. The parents want to discuss her progress and obtain information on the best way to deal with a problem at home and how to develop a particular skill.

At 3.45 p.m I set off with the hospital driver to make a home visit to talk about the progress of a child who left the unit recently. I also encourage the parents who are attempting to toilet train the boy. I arrive back at HLH just in time to catch the hospital coach back to the Maudsley and the long journey home. On the coach I discuss various problems with the students who are on placement from the IoP.

On other days, in addition to the meetings, I will see more of the children, make phone calls, dictate letters, give advice to people. I may be engaged in teaching on a course, and if at all possible work on my Ph.D which is hardly progressing. Each day is very full but varied. On the way home I do not usually work but read a novel or fall asleep on the train. I have never yet missed my train stop at Reading! In fact, I wake up every time the train slows down.

Mick cooks during the week and I cook at weekends. I talk to the family about my day, respecting confidentiality of course. I do not usually work in the evenings if I have been at Bethlem, but if I have been at the IoP I do some evening work as I am less tired and I always work at the weekends, writing reports and preparing lectures. Of course, I have to catch up with washing, shopping, mending and so forth. Mick and Sarah do a fair bit, Sarah, for example, gets paid for doing the ironing and hoovering. I usually go to bed at 11.30 p.m. after writing the instructions for the next day such as what to buy, what to eat and how to cook things. I also have to find my clothes for the following morning We usually go out two or three times a week, mostly on Tuesdays as Mick plays in a jazz band then and often on Fridays and Saturdays too. We no longer have baby sitters as Sarah and Anna are old enough to be left alone and can keep an eye on Matthew. I think it is a crazy way of life and I probably will not be able to keep it up forever but, at the moment, I cannot think of a job I would enjoy more.

In fact, I stayed in this job for two years before going to Rivermead Rehabilitation Centre and falling in love with brain injury rehabilitation.

5 Work trips to Australia, Japan, Brazil and India

I have been to Australia many times and I am an honorary professor at the University of Sydney thanks to my good friend Robyn Tate who has recently retired from there. I was unable to go to her retirement party but I sent a message to be read:

> To my dear friend and colleague, Robyn
> I have known you, Robyn for about 25 years and hold you in the highest esteem. I have completed a sabbatical with you in Sydney and you with me in Cambridge. You are one of the leading researchers of neuropsychological rehabilitation in the world. Your work is imaginative, innovative, considered, distinguished, thorough and clinically valuable. This is true not only of PsycBITE and SCRIBE, your two initiations of world wide importance, but of all the work you have completed throughout your career. You are a wonderful executive editor of our journal, Neuropsychological Rehabilitation, a superb presenter at conferences and one of my dearest friends. I remember our trip to Mallorca earlier this year with you and Michael. This was one of the best holidays ever and I cannot think of two people we would have enjoyed this with more. Long may our friendship continue and please enjoy your retirement (although my guess is you will be as busy as ever!)
> With all my love and a big hug
> Barbara

PsycBite, now known as NeuroBite standing for Neuro Behavioural Interventions and Treatment Evidence, is a database comprising all studies of cognitive, behavioural, emotional and other treatments involving survivors of acquired brain injury. It is a free, web-based resource influenced by PEDro, a Physiotherapy Evidence Database. Both NeuroBite and PEDro are free databases of thousands of randomised trials, systematic reviews and clinical practice guidelines. All trials are independently assessed for quality. These quality ratings are employed to quickly guide users to trials that are more likely to be valid and to contain sufficient information to guide clinical practice. Robyn and her colleagues were working on the studies to be entered into NeuroBite when I was on sabbatical in Australia in 2001. I was very impressed with the rigour with which each paper was evaluated before being entered into the data base.

SCRIBE is another initiative that came from Robyn's work. It stands for 'The Single-Case Reporting guideline In Behavioural intervention'. The guidelines present 26 items that authors need to address when writing about single-case experimental design (SCED) research for publication in a scientific journal. Each item is described, a rationale for its inclusion is provided, and examples of adequate reporting taken from the literature are quoted. It is recommended that SCRIBE is used by authors preparing manuscripts describing SCED research for publication, as well as journal reviewers and editors who are evaluating such manuscripts. Although the chief SCRIBE paper was published in ten journals, the main one being *Archives of Scientific Psychology* in 2016, the whole process began in 2011 when Robyn obtained a grant to invite selected people to attend a meeting in Sydney to discuss the guidelines. I was one of those people and it seemed too good an opportunity to miss. We all stayed in the wonderful Observatory Hotel in Sydney and worked hard for several days putting the guidelines together. We tidied up everything by email and the influential paper was published in 2016. On this occasion the 26 authors of the SCRIBE Statement paper were split almost 50% between men and women (12:14), with contributors from Australia, the United States of America, Canada, Spain and the United Kingdom. Why so many more women now than in decades past? It may be that psychological science has moved on from the days when women were in the minority or it may be that Australian women are more emancipated.

I'd just like to add here that I have spent many wonderful times in Australia and visited every Australian state. The country wherever you are, always seems so impressive, and I love being with Australians, perhaps especially when the results of collaborative work is as good as this turned out to be! I also ought to add how shattered I am emotionally at the damage that the terrible fires of 2019 caused and my hope is that landscapes throughout Australia will recover.

As I write this commentary at this moment I should also remind the reader, who might think I have some kind of super memory that since my very first day at Rivermead in 1979, 41 years ago, I have kept a daily diary in which I simply keep a record of what I have done each day etc. On its own it would not entertain any reader being as it is strictly factual and not at all philosophical! However, it is proving useful as a memento to which I can refer when I am being more reflective in this book

Japan is another country I have come to like although the first trip there was difficult. I went with Mick to a conference and we had to arrange many things ourselves. Few people spoke English and those that claimed to were hard to understand. Consequently, we struggled. My later trips to Japan were organised by Japanese professional people attached to conferences and other meetings, and that made life easier. The social events at this first conference during this first trip, however, were good. We met a number of people there we knew from Europe including Volker Hoemberg from Germany, Luigi (Gino) Pizzamiglio from Italy and Rohays Perry from the UK. Rohays, who was head of Psychology Journals at Psychology Press, had asked me sometime before to start a journal to be called 'Neuropsychological Rehabilitation', which I did and became editor-in-chief with Ian Robertson as deputy editor. Amazingly, the journal is still going strong, I am still the editor-in-chief after almost 30 years and Ian remains deputy editor.

Edith Kaplan from Boston was at the conference in Japan and turned out to be a real character! Over the years, at several meetings, we have spent a fair bit of time with Edith who sadly died in 2009. Here, we were all taking part in a symposium on rehabilitation which was extremely poorly attended. In fact the only people attending our talks were the other speakers and Mick!

While we were there, two of the local dignitaries took Mick and me to dinner. We were asked if we wanted a traditional Japanese meal or not. We said we did as we wanted to experience the 'real McCoy'. The food, which turned out to be a true Japanese feast of many courses, was magnificent, but we were seated on the floor Japanese style and this made things extremely difficult! Mick in particular could not get used to it and had to squirm into many different positions with his elbow on the floor while attempting to put food into his mouth with chopsticks! The two Japanese sat straight and immaculate all evening but I kept moving around and Mick ended up lying down. At the end of the evening we both struggled to stand up and staggered out of the restaurant. From then on we have never opted for Japanese style eating and have always insisted on seats! Nevertheless, we like Japanese food.

The actual venue was held in Kyoto, one of the most beautiful and historic cities in Japan. We had a chance to see the city as well as taking a trip to Nara, in the adjacent province. Nara is famous for its temples and shrines as well as the deer which are used to people and like to be fed. We fed the deer and visited the temples one of which had a fortune kiosk. We both bought a strip of paper telling us our fortunes. Mine suggested I had a highly fulfilling marriage while Mick's said something like – 'it is a pity about your marriage but it would get better'. We read each other's notes and both burst out laughing, shocking the people around us who were taking this fortune telling lark more seriously than we were.

Other trips to Japan were much easier than this one, which was spoiled in some ways because of our own naivety. Getting over this I have grown to love and respect Japan. Mick, unfortunately has not re-visited Japan and has memories only of discomfort whilst eating and total disillusion at finding out his marriage was a failure!

My closest Japanese colleague is Toshiko Watamori, a speech and language therapist who speaks and writes very good English. She was responsible for translating the Rivermead Behavioural Memory Test and still emails me with queries regarding the scoring of the test. On one trip to Japan, Toshiko took me to Hiroshima, which was very moving. Both Mick and I can remember the time of the ghastly bombing and hating the devastation and human misery it caused. We have both been lifelong supporters of nuclear disarmament and I can only say that all my worst horrors and shame were confirmed by the visit to Hiroshima.

I was impressed by the bullet trains in Japan: one stands at a designated spot on the platform, the train stops exactly where it is supposed to, and one's assigned seat is right there! The trains are both very fast and on time. Another trip was to Sapporo on the island of Hokkaido in the north of Japan. This is where the monkeys bathe in warm water. I was not there to see them, however, but was invited by a group of families of people who had survived a brain injury. After my lecture, the families wanted to talk to me and ask questions. Once again it was brought home to me how similar the problems faced by families are wherever in the world a brain injury occurs.

Toshiko has visited us in England and we have taken her to the theatre in Bury St Edmunds and in London. In Bury St Edmunds we saw *Animal Farm*. As we were seated in the front row, and there was some farmyard mud distributed to ensure realism, we all got splattered by the end of the show which, fortunately, Toshiko found very amusing. In London, we went to the Opera House to see *Madam Butterfly* which we all enjoyed immensely. However, being Japanese, Toshiko quite naturally wanted to take photos of everything and this included the stage, the audience and the ushers all of whom tried to stop her taking the photos. Eventually, Toshiko stopped. What we learned on that occasion was that we have a similar sense of humour as we watched this beautifully dressed, dignified Japanese woman defying protocol!

In a recent email to me (16 May 2020, during the coronavirus pandemic) Toshiko wrote:

> My husband temporarily moved to Nagoya from our condominium in Tokyo in early April just before the government issued the emergency state declaration asking citizens to observe self-control and not to travel across prefectural borders. The reason for this evacuation was that the state of infection has been the worst in Tokyo while it has been fairly well controlled in Nagoya. He has been staying here for 1.5 months now and it has become our new habit to walk around the neighborhood for 2–4km/day. Our daughter Akiko now works at a public health center as a veterinarian. The center she works covers the Yokohama dock where the cruise ship Diamond Princess, with 3,700 passengers, kept in quarantine to prevent spreading COVID-19, had been berthing. She was trained how to wear and remove the protective suits but luckily she was not called upon.

Another continent where I feel I have strong links is South America: my daughter, Sarah died there and my son, Matthew married a Chilean girl and lives there with my two wonderful, bilingual grandsons, Sammy and Max; and one of my two honorary 'adopted' daughters, Anita Taub, lives in Brazil (my other 'adopted' daughter being Jessica Fish). I have been to Brazil on several occasions and I am an honorary president of the Brazilian Special Interest Group in Neuropsychology.

I wrote about Brazil in my first book and described the mother's day that Sarah and I were invited to in Sao Paulo and the help Anita and her mother gave me after Sarah died. I also wrote about my hospitalisation for pneumonia in Goiania and the good treatment I received there. I know several places in the huge country of Brazil, Sarah and I spent a good holiday in Bonito after a workshop in Sao Paulo. Anita and I have been to the Pantanal and saw many hyacinth macaws. Mick and I have been to the fantastic marine wildlife reserve in Fernando de Noronha where we saw a huge number of dolphins. We have also been to the Amazon twice, to Salvador, Recife, Paraty and, of course, to Rio de Janeiro. I was ill the first time we went to Rio, we had just visited the Amazon and I think I caught something there. I had a lecture to give in Rio but spent most of the time in bed in the hotel room while Mick explored the city by himself. The medical people in Rio thought I might have developed malaria and kept asking me 'How is your belly?' I was taking antimalarial tablets and knew I didn't have malaria. The illness cleared up after a few days. I went to Rio again several years later with Anita, stayed at The Copocabana Hotel, visited Christ the Redeemer statue, swam a great deal and had a good time. However, I know Sao Paulo better and I am impressed by the amazing and excellent restaurants there.

Another Brazilian city I have visited is Belo Horizonte as that is where my friend and colleague Fabricia Loschiavo lives. I did a two-day workshop on memory there in 2014 and afterwards I was treated to a stay in a beautiful city, Ouro Preto, 100 kilometres from Belo Horizonte, with Fabricia and her friends. We were booked in to the lovely Solar de Rosario Hotel where I stayed in the superior suite and was treated like royalty.

The year before that, on my birthday, Fabricia had sent me a video of her singing Happy Birthday with her little dog, Boneca, barking in time to the tune. It was the funniest birthday card I have ever received.

The photo on page 33 was taken on yet another visit to Brazil where I spoke at the Brazilian congress of Neuropsychology. From left to right, the people are Eliane Miotto (a good friend from the University of Sao Paulo), Anita Taub, me, Fabricia Loschiavo and Renata Ávila. We are all officials of the Brazilian special interest group in neuropsychology. As I write in May 2020, I should be preparing to go to Recife next week to give a workshop with Fabricia but this has been cancelled because of the coronavirus.

Fabricia and I have an edited book (just published), in Portuguese (Fabricia has translated the chapters written in English). In fact, she was the driving force behind all of this. It came about because of my model published in 2002 'Towards a comprehensive model of cognitive rehabilitation' (Wilson 2002). The model was to show people working in brain injury not only the complexity but also the steps to take when planning rehabilitation. Much of Fabricia's work is with neuropsychiatric patients and she adapted the model for that group. This paper was published in 2018 (Loschiavo-Alvares, Wilson & Fish 2018). The next step was for Fabricia to expand this further into a book. She persuaded me to co-edit this with her and I was very impressed with her drive and enthusiasm.

Another friend and colleague I have mentioned is Eliane Miotto. She completed her PhD in London with Robin Morris and that is when I first met her. She then returned to Brazil and is a senior person in neuropsychology at the University of Sao Paulo. Eliane and her husband, Elias, have entertained me several times in Sao Paulo and we have also met up in London at meetings. They are always very gracious hosts.

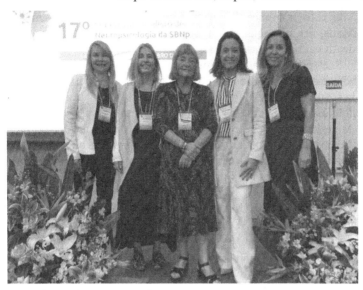

Figure 5.1 Barbara in Brazil with officers of the Brazilian Neuropsychological Society.

India is a yet another country I have visited on several occasions. I often say it is both wonderful and awful but, fortunately, the wonderful parts outweigh the awful parts. I have good friends in India and love the hospitality, the food, and the colourful life of the streets. However, I don't like the poverty, the shanty towns and the state of some of the dogs I see in the street. My first trip to India was in 2006 to attend a conference in Chennai (formerly Madras). Anne-Lise Christensen from Copenhagen was there and we decided to go on a trip to the Gold Triangle afterwards. I first met Anne-Lise in 1985 when she opened the Centre for Rehabilitation of Brain Injury (CBRI). Anne-Lise had actually invited Freda Newcombe, (a neuropsychologist famous for her work on the long-term follow-up of soldiers who had sustained a brain injury in the Second World War), to go to the opening of the new centre but Freda (who died in 2001) could not go and asked me to step in. I then went to the ten-year and twenty-year anniversaries of the centre. Anne-Lise was a friend of Luria's and published a number of texts advocating Luria's approach to neuropsychological assessment. Sadly, she died in February 2018. I had an email from Frank Humle, the director of the CBRI and Lise Lambek, Anne-Lise's secretary, saying:

This is to announce that Anne-Lise passed away Sunday morning. Mads, her son, tells that it was as undramatic and as peaceful as death can be in certain cases.

She spent the last 15 months at the nursing home in Adelaide where an empathetic and competent staff has taken good care of her, and made the difficult end to a long and exciting life as tolerable as possible. She was obviously pleased with life till the end. Anne-Lise has donated her body to the Anatomical Institute, so there will be no funeral service. We will miss her, but she will be in our hearts forever – and we will carry on her outstanding work at the CRBI. Best, Frank and Lise.

Back to the trip to the Golden Triangle. This comprises three cities in the north west of India, Delhi, Agra and Jaipur. We also added on a visit to Ranthambore, a tiger reserve. Seeing the Taj Mahal in Agra was special and as stunning as expected, although, for me, the highlight was Ranthambore. The reserve was very beautiful and we saw many antelope and other animals but we did not see any tigers. In fact I did not see tigers in the wild until a visit to Bandhavgarh several years later. The one problem encountered during this first tour was that Anne-Lise did not like spicy food! Every place we stayed had to do a special menu for her!

I have some superb memories of many other Indian trips but will just mention a few here. In 2011, I went there again to receive the Ramon Y. Cahal award for distinguished contributions to neuropsychiatry (from the International Neuropsychiatric Association) but on an even later visit in 2013, presenting a workshop with colleagues in Kolkata, I arranged a trip to Bandhavgarh, a tiger reserve, where I heard there was a good chance of seeing tigers. Before the workshop, I went to stay with Jwala Narayan and her family in Bangalore where I was very well treated in their lovely house. We also went to a delightful concert in the city. I told Jwala's father that after the conference I was going to Bandhavgarh, and he told me to tell the guide he would receive a good tip if we saw tigers. This was to turn out to be a valuable piece of advice as we will see.

Meanwhile, the conference in Kolkata was good. My friend and honorary 'adopted' son Jon Evans was there, so was Narinder, my British-Indian colleague and good friends from India including Jwala Narayanan and Urvashi Shah from Mumbai. After the workshop, I had to take a late train from Kolkata to Katni, a town in Madhya Pradesh in the middle of India where I was to make the connection by car to Bandhavgarh. I had booked a first-class sleeper on the train and several friends came to the station to wish me a safe journey. I know that Narinder and his wife Ritu were worried about me travelling alone and, to be honest, I was a little worried too. This was just after a terrible gang rape in Delhi which was on all the news channels.

Well, the train was about three hours late so we all just waited at the railway station and that was an adventure in itself. Not only was the station absolutely packed, it was also full of porters with impossibly high loads on their barrels, which, having no brakes, the porters simply yelled at people to get out of their way. In addition, there were rats everywhere. It was an incredible scene hard to imagine for someone who has not been to India. Eventually, the train arrived very late at night and my friends helped me to settle into my compartment. This wasn't the luxurious first class I was expecting, but it wasn't too bad. There were four bunks in the compartment, three were taken by men and I was in the fourth. None of the men spoke. I tried to make my luggage secure and settled down for the night. The train to Katni took 19 hours. I realised the next day that not only was I the only white woman on the train, I was the only woman travelling alone!

I watched rural India go past feeling a little apprehensive. About one hour before reaching Katni, one of the men in the carriage asked me where I was getting off, I told him and he wanted to know if I had a driver waiting. I said I did and he suggested I phone the driver to tell him what carriage I was in and he would wait at the right spot on the platform. I found the number of the driver and phoned him on my British mobile phone. Unfortunately, he did not speak English. The helpful Indian man said he would phone and explain in Hindi. He did this and the driver was waiting at exactly the right spot when I left the train. I was expecting Katni to be a quiet little town but no, it was bustling, busy and overcrowded like any other place in India.

The drive to Bandhavgarh seemed to take forever but eventually the driver delivered me to a good hotel late at night. There were staff there to welcome me and I slept well. The next morning was my first game drive. I said to the man that there would be a good tip if I saw tigers. He was supposed to follow a certain route but then said he would go off the route as there was a tiger nearby. We soon saw a female tigress lying in the grass. I was pleased but the guide was nervous as he had left his allotted route (where I would not have seen the tiger). He said he had to get back to his route and went down a little path. As he did so, a huge male tiger ambled past very close to our vehicle! I took some video footage and still shots. The tiger sprayed a nearby tree and then sauntered off into the bushes. I was so excited and pleased. I did tip well and silently thanked Jwala's father for giving me this information. I was also a little cross as I would never have seen tigers without this offer of a good tip and visitors should not have to do that. Would Anne-Lise and I have seen them in Ranthambore had we offered a reward? We didn't know then that it could be the secret weapon.

The next year I was back in India again, in Chennai for another workshop partly funded, once more, by the World Federation of NeuroRehabilitation's flying faculty. After the workshop I was to give the Gopalakrishna Endowment Lecture entitled 'The art and science of neurorehabilitation'. Gopalakrishna is a medical doctor specialising in infectious diseases. His wife had founded an orphanage about one hour's drive from the city and Mick and I were invited to visit. We were unsure what to expect or what to take as a present. We decided on some drawing materials and coloured pencils which we left with the teacher in the school at the orphanage.

A female member of staff was our guide and took us to 2 of the 20 or so houses which formed the complex. Each home comprised several children of different ages ranging from about 2 years of age to 16 or 17. There was a 'mother' in charge of each house. We did not see many toys or furnishings but the children seemed far more adjusted than the children in orphanages I had seen in the UK. Our children seem to need to cling on to adults and want lots of attention and affection whereas the Indian children were 'normal'. They behaved appropriately and did not cling on to us. We were told that when the children came to school leaving age, they were helped to find jobs; later they also stayed in touch with the 'mothers'. We learned that the 'mothers' were always unmarried and employed at the age of 17 or 18 years. Their main job was to love the children in their care. I was impressed. In one house we were told that the 'mother' was retiring the following day. I asked where she would go and was told that she would live with one of her departed grown up 'children'. I was even more impressed. Just before we left, the guide said that the retiring mother was a bereaved parent, one of her 'children' had died in an accident and one had died through suicide. I asked the guide to explain in her own language that I was also a bereaved parent after which the two of us hugged each other as bereaved parents do. I left the orphanage complex with respect for what was happening there. Before this meeting we went on a trip to the wonderful Mahabalipuram, a city in Tamil Nadu and a UNESCO world heritage site. I have been there twice. It has the best bas relief that I have ever seen. The rock carvings date from the seventh and eighth centuries. The first time I went was after an earlier conference in Chennai when my friend, Jwala, came from Bangalore with a driver to take me there. I was astonished at the wonder of it all. These are a few of the many wonderful trips I have taken in association with work and some more will be described in a later chapter.

6   Jordan, my last trip with Sarah

Until she died, and while Mick suffered with an arthritic knee before having an artificial knee implanted in 1998), Sarah was my main travelling companion. One of the best trips we took was to Jordan. We left just after Christmas in 1997 and were there for New Year 1998. Matthew drove us to Heathrow on 27 December, we spent the night at The Holiday Inn and left on 28 December. Sarah was a little downhearted as she had just separated from Jez and they had decided to get a divorce. They had undergone seven years of unsuccessful treatment for infertility and I believe this had taken a toll. In three attempts, Sarah didn't keep any of the implanted embryos for more than a week. If she had a baby, of course, she would never had gone to Peru and the white water rafting trip in May 2000 and would not have died there.

We left for Amman, the capital of Jordan, the following day and met up with our group from Explore Worldwide that I have travelled with on a number of occasions. Being mother and daughter, Sarah and I shared a room throughout. We loved the entire trip and enjoyed the group; it was less quarrelsome than the Madagascar group I describe elsewhere.

After a night in Amman, we visited Jerash, just 30 miles away in the north of the country. Jerash is famous for its Roman ruins and is one of the best preserved Roman sites in the world. For this reason it is sometimes called the Pompeii of the Middle East. Jerash is, in fact, much older than the Roman period, with the earliest evidence of settlement in Jerash being a Neolithic site known as Tal Abu Sowan, where rare human remains dating to around 7500 BC were uncovered. Jerash flourished during the Greek and Roman periods until the eighth century AD, when an earthquake in Galilee, destroyed large parts of it. Later earthquakes caused additional damage. Among the Roman ruins is Hadrian's Arch, this is the same Hadrian that built our wall between England and Scotland.

From Jerash we visited Mount Nebo, where Moses is supposed to have seen the promised land. From the summit, one can see the valley of Jordan, the city of Jericho and sometimes Jerusalem on a clear day. This was followed by the highlight of the tour, a two-day visit to Petra known as 'the rose red city, half as old as time'. I thought that maybe Petra would be a disappointment given we had heard so much about it, but it was far from that. We approached the city on foot through a narrow canyon called Al Siq, initially not much can be seen, then slowly the famous building known as the Treasury comes into view. At first a tiny part of it is seen and then, gradually, more and more of the building appears. It is breathtaking. The whole city is wonderful; founded by the Nabateans 300 BC, it is truly an incredible place. Our group comprised mostly younger people who were all for climbing to the city at the top on foot. Sarah joined them. I decided I would hire one of the guides with a donkey and ride up. I was told it would cost the equivalent of 8 pounds sterling which at the time I thought expensive but by the time the poor donkey had carried me all the way up with the guide walking beside us, I thought I had not been charged enough for the effort! I talked to the guys en route and wondered why I did not see any women. It became obvious the women were hidden away and their inferior status became even clearer when I was offered so many camels for Sarah to be married to one of the locals. No doubt this was meant as a joke but I thought it was a bit too close to the bone to be comfortable with. The men were an interesting group to talk to, nevertheless, and one guy had a broad cockney accent! It turned out he had spent many years working in London.

After our stay in the beautiful city of Petra, we travelled south to Wadi Rum, in the desert, and camped with the Bedouins. We arrived on New Year's Eve. I knew that I was likely to get an OBE (order of the British Empire) in the Queen's New Year's honours list as two months earlier I received a letter from the then prime minister Tony Blair. The letter arrived while I was at a meeting in Italy and was waiting for me when I returned home. It read something like this: 'The PM had it in mind to award me this honour. If he recommended this to the Queen would I accept and was I happy with receiving the OBE for services to medical rehabilitation?' I was also asked not to tell anyone about the letter and the recommendation. I was in shock, uncertain what to do wondering whether or not to accept. I knew my father would not approve as he would not let us stand up for the national anthem (which we would have to do if I went to Buckingham Palace to receive the award). I also knew that some people like David Bowie had refused to be honoured. On the other hand, Mick wanted me to accept saying it would be good for rehabilitation, so I wrote a letter saying I would accept the award if it were to be offered. I also accepted the reason for being given the award although in retrospect I should have changed 'medical rehabilitation' to 'psychological rehabilitation'. With the letter sent, I heard nothing more and conjectured whether or not the letter had gone missing in the post. Anyway, I did not mention this to anyone in the Explore group visiting Jordan. Sarah knew of course and had been instrumental in sending the letter to the honours awards committee, after obtaining letters from various people who knew me including families of brain injured people I had helped. One of the people visiting Jordan with us was a priest who arranged a service to celebrate the New Year. Sarah and I did not go being atheists but we told him it was a good thing to do. We had a New Year's Eve party in the desert that night with the Bedouins.

The following day we phoned home partly to wish everyone 'Happy New Year' and partly to find out about the OBE. Mick told me that I had indeed been awarded an OBE and he had been on television, on Look East, to do an interview. I had been wanted but wasn't available so Mick had found a photo of me with a camel taken on another trip and this was shown on screen as he was interviewed while doing some ironing. He had wanted to make a point about men sharing the housework but nobody seemed to notice and it was never commented on. At dinner that night Sarah announced my award to the group and we had an impromptu party under the stars with the Bedouins. Thus my receiving the award was to some extent celebrated. I had to go to the palace later in the year for the investiture and will say more about that soon.

We enjoyed our stay in Wadi Rum; I always like deserts as their scenery and geology are intriguing. This particular desert is in a valley cut into sandstone with granite rock surrounding it. Like other places in Jordan, Wadi Rum has been inhabited by many human cultures since prehistoric times. The Nabataeans who founded Petra were here too and left rock paintings, graffiti and temples. Those readers who know about T.E. Lawrence (of 'Lawrence of Arabia' fame) may have heard about Wadi Rum because he visited the area several times during the Arab Revolt of 1917–18. Our group explored the area by a four wheeled vehicle unlike the horses that Lawrence used.

Our next trip was to Aqaba and the Red Sea where we were rather lazy but we did go snorkelling. The city was disappointing with building sites and rubble but the reef was beautiful. It was almost vertical rather than horizontal like the Great Barrier Reef in Queensland, Australia, and I remember being surprised at this. We did see plenty of fish, though. Aqaba, the only coastal city in Jordan, is in fact very close to Eilat in Israel, a city I had visited some years before.

We had one more stop in Jordan before setting off back to Amman and home. This was to the Dead Sea, the lowest point on earth. One floats there as it is extremely salty and almost impossible to swim in or to drown! Again, I had been there before but on the Israeli side. I did not find the Dead Sea an exciting place to be, it was not my favourite place in either of the two countries. We travelled home safely and with no further adventures.

Soon after arriving home, I received a letter asking which date I wanted to go to London for the investiture of the OBE. I chose a date in May that year, knowing I would not be abroad then. I was told I could take three visitors with me so chose, Mick, Sarah and Rosie who was 10 years old at the time. We decided to splash out and stay at the Savoy hotel in London, a famous hotel near to Buckingham Palace and we had a special parking ticket to allow us to enter Buckingham Palace. We drove to London in Mick's slightly beaten Mazda MX6 and parked at the Savoy. We had booked two adjoining rooms, one for us and one for Sarah and Rosie. We swam in the pool and had dinner there. At breakfast the next day we told some of the staff we were going to the palace and were advised to walk but we wanted to drive and use our special parking ticket. Some of this is reported in the first memoirs book but in less detail. Here I quote from the first book.

> We had an interesting day. Prince Charles was giving the awards that day and we were told that was good because the Queen gave each person 15 seconds whereas Charles gave everyone 30 seconds. The guests were led to one room and the people receiving awards were given a lesson by the Prince's equerry, a tall man in military uniform, who had to show the females how to curtsey! We were told to walk in one way, curtsey and walk forward. When the Prince shook our hand that was the signal to leave and we should back out before departing in the opposite direction. I waited in a queue between a woman getting an award for services to marriage counselling and another receiving an award for services to the National Trust. I liked the awards because they were not academic but given for public service. It seemed a good thing to me.
>
> When it was my turn to speak to Charles, he said to me, 'So you come from that famous place?' I didn't know if he meant Cambridge or The Oliver Zangwill Centre or what so I said, I work in Cambridge with people who have survived a brain injury. He asked if we had made any progress to which I said yes, but we needed more money. 'Oh, the perennial problem,' said the Prince and put out his hand – my signal to go. I don't think I should

have mentioned money! I am not sure how much the OBE has helped rehabilitation but some people are impressed with me having an OBE. It stands for Order of the British Empire and, of course, we no longer have an empire so it sounds a misnomer. Sometimes I get letters addressed to Professor Obe!' (Wilson 2020, pp. 89–90).

7   Present time

Brexit and the coronavirus; and a look back to early marriage when we lived in Suffolk and Essex and neuropsychology was not even thought of

I am at home and have been at home for a total of eight weeks because of the coronavirus that has struck the world. This is not just the biggest disaster that has hit me in my lifetime (other than Sarah dying, of course), it is the biggest catastrophe that has attacked the whole of mankind for centuries! I'm trying not to feel sorry for myself as I remember completing the first book of memoirs, of which this is the second, just at the time when the British cast their vote overwhelmingly in favour of a Tory government and its support for Brexit. So we were left in the air, as it were, at the end of the first book having lost on Brexit a second time – and more convincingly. From one angle our arguments expressed in Book One against Brexit now look plaintive and irrelevant. Except that, from a different angle, another story seems to be unfolding from the viral lockdown, which suggests that leaving Europe could have been a very bad thing to do in the light of the need for individual countries to get closer together in their fight against a world pandemic. Trying to go it alone, as the UK and USA seem to want might be disastrous in any fight against such a giant opponent as coronavirus. Not that the countries in the European Union did much collaborative fighting against the virus when the time came to oppose the pandemic initially! Nevertheless, the British record for fighting coronavirus has not been good. In fact, it's looking like being one of the worst in comparison with the rest of the world except for Trump's USA, and maybe Brazil which is catching up at speed!

In the *Guardian* of 9 May 2020 Heather Stewart quotes Lisa Nandy, who was one of the candidates for leader of the Labour Party and now shadow foreign secretary, when she argued that the Conservative government's 'go it alone' approach left Britain unable to prepare for coronavirus. Nandy calls our approach 'exceptionalism', taking on an isolationist route where Britain in particular champions the idea of a small island nation that would punch above its weight without stopping to think about how we're going to exert power ... What we've learned in this pandemic, is that the global Britain approach that was supposed to put Britain first, has ended up putting us among the last'. Nandy went on to say, 'Britain was one of those countries where a myth of "exceptionalism" had taken hold, leading to "an enormous divergence" in the way the outbreak had been tackled, creating problems for citizens and businesses.' As I write this a newsflash has just come on to announce that deaths in Britain have gone up by 468!

I am left wondering why it is that Mick and I feel, in the deepest part of ourselves, deeper than the immediate misery of the nation's lockdown, a tiny bit buoyant? I think it's because we know that when this disaster is over things will never be the same again. Many of our relatives and friends have expressed similar feelings, pointing to the many acts of kindness and expressions of social responsibility communicated by neighbours, shop assistants and people in the street. Will this pandemic really lead to the end of capitalism and materialism? And the other thing is that people have been noticing that nature itself is looking and sounding much better. Does this mean that eventually David Attenborough might live to see some of the global changes he has been urging the world to make? Also, on the news today they have been commiserating with adolescents who were about to take exams when coronavirus struck. I feel so sorry for them, they don't know which way to turn and they are frightened of what the future may hold for them in terms of higher education and eventual careers.

We didn't have any of this in the early 1960s. Mick remembers that at the end of his teacher training course the college gymnasium walls were covered with hundreds and hundreds of job offers. Mind you, he also remembers his first month's pay, which was £34.00!

I've just checked on the Internet, the average house price in the 1960s was £2,530. We bought our first house in Brook Street, Colchester in 1965, when Sarah was a little over 2 years old, Anna was just over a year and I was pregnant with Matthew who was to be born in that house. We were a very close and busy family, Mick working seven days a week: his weekends were spent in lesson preparation for the coming week; which was an intense activity as he always aimed to make every single lesson entertaining and demanding for the pupils! And he helped me with such things as nappy washing, etc. There were only washable nappies available in those years! All three lots were washed in the bath and hung to dry on the very long washing line. Oh, and Mick also took up vegetable growing – which remained with him all our married life until about six years ago when we moved into a town house in Bury St Edmunds. I was keeping my mind active with various evening classes and cooking which I have always enjoyed plus trying to be a good mother to the children. I read to them, took them out regularly to the zoo, the park and did other things I thought would be good for them. I must say, though, that I was frustrated at not having a 'proper' job.

So there we were, a neat little family with our roles clearly defined and tending towards the traditional despite our socialist sympathies and hippy outlook. We were certainly hard-working. We did go to the pub once a week – at the top of the street where we met up with building workers who Mick had met when doing holiday jobs on the building sites; and then there was Mick's family, his mum and dad, three sisters and a brother all living in Ipswich 18 miles due east. We had two great friends, Neil and Ann Dean, who lived in Ipswich and two more, Mike and Sue Crooks, who lived in Capel St Mary next door to Stratford St Mary situated half way between Ipswich and Colchester.

Stratford St Mary was a focal point for Mick before I met him, a place he knew well because one of its inhabitants was Ida Hughes Stanton, who lived in a delightful but run-down thatched residence know as Weaver's Cottage with her companion Don Nevard, who was a jazz pianist. Ida was a striking bohemian figure from the 1930s who knew lots of celebrities from that era – which impressed a lot of working class kids from Ipswich and Colchester, interested principally in jazz and art, who used to meet at Ida's to listen to jazz records, swim and punt in the river and end up drinking in Dedham.

I grew to love Stratford St Mary, so much a part Constable country, situated at a bend in the River Stour where you can still see Le Talbooth pub and restaurant, which was described by Daniel Defoe in *Moll Flanders* one of the very first novels ever to have been written. This was in the early eighteenth century. Whenever we had visitors we would take them on a Constable country tour. The first stop was to go to a little wooden bridge over the River Stour at Stratford and take a photograph looking down the river. It's the exact spot where John Constable painted *Stratford Mill* a painting which hangs in the National Gallery and for which it is impossible to buy a postcard or a print from the Gallery's shop. There are loads of *The Haywain* of course, perhaps Constable's most famous painting. I belong to the National Gallery's support membership and I didn't get any joy from them when I enquired why there was no reproduction of *Stratford Mill*. So, if you want to see it you'll have to go the National Gallery. Or maybe I can get a really nice photo taken to accompany this story? Even better, if we can make a comparison of the painting and a modern photo? That way we might be able to see what Constable does to change a site into a masterpiece?

One of our visitors much later when we were living in Flempton – it must have been in the early 2000s – near Bury St Edmunds, and when Mick was truly retired from publishing, was Elizabeth Warrington. Her important contributions in theoretical understanding of neuropsychological disorders, as Professor of Clinical Neuropsychology at the National Hospital, Queen Square, are renowned internationally. She came to visit as she was particularly interested in gardens and had a good garden at home in London. At that time, our garden was about one acre in size. Elizabeth seemed to appreciate it and, of course, we took her on the Constable country tour. This included Mick rowing us in a tiny boat a quarter way up the river and we believe this, too, was enjoyed by Elizabeth.

Sitting here at home on 22 May 2020 and not being able to go out because of the coronavirus lockdown, I am able to escape back in time through writing this memoir and I make no excuse for the inevitable name dropping that occurs in the text. After all, if you cannot drop names when writing an autobiography whenever can you? This next name is, in Mick's estimation, *un nom par excellence*, and the story goes like this.

We were staying at Mike and Sue's place in Capel St Mary one weekend when Mike informed us that on the Saturday night we had been invited to a party to be held in one of the bungalows recently built in the village. For some reason, and I don't know why, Mick and I turned up at the bungalow without Mike and Sue, who came later. We knocked on the door and it was opened by a smiling Bobby Robson, ex-manager of Ipswich Town Football team and now manager of England! I didn't recognise him immediately but Mick suddenly went very quiet and perhaps a bit pale. Anyway, this warm and friendly man asked us our names, drew us in to the front room and asked us what we would like to drink. Mick was able to whisper to me that the guy was Bobby Robson who, in the opinion of many experts was the best manager England ever had! The night at the party progressed smoothly with Bobby being the main person who looked after our well-being. We were impressed with his kindness, modesty, and above all his sense of fun! He didn't talk football all evening but was most interested in listening to us and talking about his brother, who was obviously a hero of Bobby's, who had remained a miner all his life. Mick said later that Bobby made us feel ten feet tall – and added that's what he did with his football teams. He was certainly one of the most loved, admired and distinguished managers England has ever had. Just to give you some idea of his reputation, indeed his fame, I quote a small section from Wikipedia:

> In March 2011, The East Coast train operating company named one of its first class locomotives, Sir Bobby Robson. In December 2011 the Port of Tyne authority named its new work boat the Sir Bobby Robson. In 2012 a statue of Robson was unveiled at St. James Park football stadium. On 16 July 2013, marking the 150th anniversary of the Football Association, the FA designated 10 August as the *Sir Bobby Robson National Football Day*, as a day to celebrate the national game.

Just one more person from those days, and this is Venice Manley, someone who died penniless, having spent her last few years in a poky flat in Finchley, London, where she had to share a toilet situated on the landing with several others. Despite having found fame in the music world she never found fortune. Mick's connection with Venice was via Ida Hughes Stanton in earlier days as Venice was a major character in the Ipswich jazz crowd. Later in our marriage I also got to know Venice and coincidentally, at her memorial service held in a boat on the River Thames, I bumped into an ex-patient of the Oliver Zangwill Centre, who was attending the memorial service because he had been in her Georgian choir. To give you an idea of Venice, her history, her character, her beauty and her talent, I am going to quote from a tribute to her written by Helen Chadwick after Venice died in a London hospital 16 years ago and published on the Internet (Helen Chadwick, downloaded from the Internet on 22 May 2020):

> Venice sang classical music and Eastern European folk songs, spirituals and her own songs. She taught singing to individuals, theatre companies and choirs. She worked in Canada, America, Germany, Holland and France. In the last five years of her life she ran Maspinzeli, The London Georgian Choir. She had a luminous presence. She sang in the acapella group known as Kite. As a baby she had been left by her parents with slightly reluctant neighbours for a year. But her parents never came back and when, at the age of eleven, she was run over by a bus and lost half her leg, they adopted her. She ran away the day she legally could and became a traveller of sorts. With her partner she became involved with the rights of the travellers in Ireland and later set up and taught in a Montessori school for their children with money she raised from Yul Brynner (whose mother was a gypsy) and the Beatles.

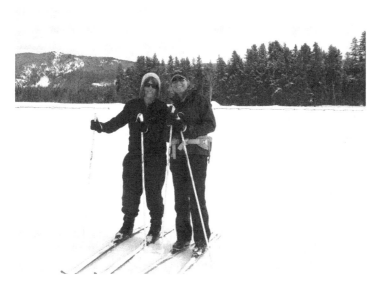

Figure 7.1 Barbara skiing in Colorado. We learned to ski cross-country in Colorado. Mick was jealous because I was better than him. He said it was because I have a lower centre of gravity. Ha-ha!

Her childhood dream was to be a dancer, but after the accident it was singing which became her passion, though she remained a graceful mover and dancer all her life and many people had no idea that she was physically disabled. She loved it when maxi skirts were the fashion as they covered her artificial leg.

Much later in life she finally found and met her birth father. He adored her and until his death this father was a great source of love for her. Even in hospital, when she was dying, at the age of 69, she remained an entertainer. Friends and singers came to visit her from far and near, the table was full of flowers and cards, and people came away laughing from her stories and antics, even though she was in terrible pain. A few days before she died we sang together many of her favourite songs.

Mick can add two stories from the late 1950s. One involves Venice's expulsion from grammar school at the age of 13. She was guilty of tying toilet rolls round the door knobs of classroom doors in a classroom quadrangle; and less than two years since she had lost half her leg, she had to walk down the school hallway to the stage where she had to hand in her school scarf and hat, turn round and march out of the hall and out of the school gate accompanied by a posse of girls.

Mick's own story involved punting down the River Stour, to Weaver's House with Venice, Mike and himself after a night's drinking in Dedham. It must have been in 1960, a year before I met him. As they approached their landing Venice stood up in the boat which in consequence tipped over throwing them all in the water from which they drunkenly swam to the river bank, Venice laughing loudest, and Mick worrying whether her artificial leg would fill with water.

8 My first day at Rivermead Rehabilitation Centre

In the first book, I explained how I found my feet at Rivermead Rehabilitation Centre (RRC) in 1979 and realised on my first day that I would stay in brain injury rehabilitation for the rest of my career, which I most certainly have done. As readers will know, I keep a work journal which I started after my first day at RRC. I had no real idea what was expected of me in this new job, having worked, since qualifying as a clinical psychologist, with children having developmental learning disabilities, many of whom also had severe self-injurious behaviour. I thought that if *I* did not know what to expect, this would also be true of other clinical psychologists and therefore I would write about the job so others could discover what was entailed in brain injury rehabilitation. This became my very first daily journal and much of this chapter is based on my initial thoughts and observations as initially expressed in that journal. (The comments in italics are my observations from the present day.)

Monday October 1st 1979. I started my new job today, at RRC in Oxford. When I arrived at 8.40 a.m, I met Dr Rushworth, the consultant in charge. She introduced me to one of the speech therapists, Helen, who showed me to my room. The room is big and spacious but gloomy. Apparently it is soon to be decorated. The room is also cold as the central heating has not yet been turned on. There is a one bar electric fire attached to the wall; this heats my desk but not much else. I met the head speech therapist, Anne Hankey and a research psychologist, Greg, who was doing some research on stroke patients.

From 9.00–10.00 am I unpacked books and papers and sorted out the cupboard containing test materials. I found most materials I will probably need in the near future, the WAIS, the Wechsler Memory Scale, the Benton Visual Retention Test, Raven's Progressive Matrices and the Rey-Osterreith Complex Figure. I found, too, various reading scales, personality questionnaires, and vocational guidance forms. There was an aphasia test and a memory battery I had never heard of before. I would really like to order the complete Luria neuropsychological test battery and will ask May Davidson (*the then district psychologist*) about ordering it.

Having spent an hour sorting things out, I braced myself to go and face more people at the centre. My first stop was to the secretaries' office to ask about ordering lunch and how the internal mail system worked. I ordered lunch and paid 40 pence to the cook (*how cheap that sounds now!*) I then sent my various forms to the personnel officer at The Nuffield Hospital. My next call was to the workshop building where patients do their occupational therapy (OT). I found Stephanie, senior OT, whom I had met before on a visit to RRC the previous month and a basic grade OT who had also just started today. They were obviously busy so I did not stay but went back to my room. I started to read a hand out on the work of a clinical psychologist when Jane Moore, a junior doctor, came in and asked if I would see a young 16 year old lad who had been involved in a motorcycle accident. He was causing difficulties for the staff and they wanted a treatment programme for him. I said I would see him and read his notes. By then it was 10.30 a.m and I went over to the common room for coffee and to meet more people.

My next job was to find the ward where the notes were kept, introduce myself to the staff nurse and borrow the notes in order to read what had happened to the 16 year old lad. He had been involved in a motorcycle accident five months earlier and had been unconscious for 10 days. He had sustained a basal skull fracture and showed signs of brain stem damage. He was admitted to RRC 8 weeks previously and had progressed well since then. Now he was having behaviour problems. I needed to speak to the lad and to the staff who were complaining about his behaviour. I found him in the OT block and arranged to see him straightaway, for half an hour. He did not admit to any problems except to say he was worried about the up coming court case that was happening because of the accident. I decided that I could not design a treatment programme until I had spoken to the staff and worked out the antecedents, the actual behaviour and the consequences of this (an ABC chart, in fact). I could then obtain a baseline and consider an extinction programme with positive reinforcement or a shaping procedure or maybe a token economy programme. I took the young man back to OT and wrote some notes on him.

Each Monday a staff meeting is held with the OTs, physiotherapists and speech therapists. I went along to get to know people. Stephanie ran the meeting, she went through the names of various patients and the other staff reported back. After hearing one of the physiotherapists say, rather doubtfully, that one patient was improving, I wondered how improvement was evaluated. I decided to ask about that as it might be something for which we could work out a systematic procedure, unless that had already been done, of course. Someone else said that one of the patients could not tie his shoelaces and I was unsure whether this was because of a physical or a cognitive/spatial problem. If the latter then Janet Carr's method of teaching the learning disabled children at Hilda Lewis House might work using two different coloured laces and a backward chaining procedure. (*As I write this in 2020, Janet Carr's obituary has just appeared in the Guardian and the Psychologist: this wonderful woman died in her sleep on 17 March just before her 93rd birthday and was well known for her studies of people with Down's Syndrome. She was an inspiration to me and to many others*).

The other point that interested me during the meeting was a discussion about a patient with possible apraxia who could walk without help but who said she could not move her leg. One of the physios said it was more usual for a patient to do an incorrect movement of the leg than to say she could not move her leg (when the patient obviously could move her leg or she would have been unable to walk). I decided I needed to see the patient and find out what was happening. I wish I were more experienced in neuropsychology as it is one thing teaching it to students as I had been doing at the Institute of Psychiatry and another thing to work on the practical side with patients. The meeting finished at 12.30 and I went to read some of Luria's testing manual until lunch at 1.00 p.m.

From 1.30 until 4.30 p.m I was with the OTs and the patients apart from a 15 minute tea break at 3.15 p.m. Sue Whiting, the sector OT was very helpful and explained the Bobarth method to me. This is a way of encouraging stroke patients with a hemiplegia and some patients with a TBI (a traumatic brain injury) to use their affected sides. Sue Whiting is so interesting to listen to and a good teacher as well. I found the afternoon useful especially when observing the woman the physios had spoken about in the morning. As well as being able to walk, she can talk reasonably well although she has some problems with word finding. She can also read but seems unable to match things according to the OTs. I saw her for a while in OT and she was unable to name some pictures I showed her. Then Wendy, one of the OTs, asked the patient to make a cup of tea. This was so difficult for the patient, she could not fill the kettle, get things ready or pour the milk. I felt she needed a step-by-step procedure worked out for her to follow, either by reading the steps or through being taken through each step separately with a backward chaining procedure. I feel I must do a thorough neuropsychological assessment with her and work out some teaching strategies. She is a fascinating woman and aware of her problems. She frequently laughed at her mistakes while saying that she used not to be as silly as this (*like many brain injured people she blames herself for the mistakes rather than the brain damage*).

When I asked her to name the pictures, she said that one part of her wanted to give the right answer and the other part the wrong one. I find that thought provoking; it is as if the right hemisphere knows that the left has misnamed the picture but cannot do anything about it. She read the digits 1, 2, 3 correctly but much more slowly than she read single words. I wonder how she would read 'one, two, three'? I believe she has a disconnection syndrome as Geschwind describes and I hope to spend some time investigating that. Just before I left the OTs at 4.30 p.m., one of the secretaries phoned to ask me to meet her so she could show me my pigeon hole and how to pick up the internal post. I did that and found a welcome note from Beryl, the secretary at the Warneford Hospital, where the district psychology department is based, and providing details about the area departmental meeting at the Warneford tomorrow. I realised this would clash with a ward round at RRC but thought it would be good to meet other psychologists in the area.

After returning to my room, which is in the same block as the speech therapist and research psychologist, I saw Anne, the senior speech therapist, who asked if anyone had spoken to me about the woman with the possible apraxia. I said I had seen her briefly and would be arranging to do an assessment and a treatment programme with her soon.

Just before leaving, the young doctor came in again to ask me to see a young man who needed to lose weight. This was Derek (not his real name) that I talk about in the earlier book. Initially referred for help with his weight problem, I ended up treating him both for his weight problem and for his acquired dyslexia. I left at 5.00 p.m. That evening I reread Geschwind's important paper on Disconnection Syndromes (Geschwind 1965). *I actually met Norman Geschwind, a lovely and important man, at a meeting on reading* disorders in Greece in 1984, two months before he died prematurely at the age of 58 years. I have a photo of the two of us taken in September 1984 about two months before he died. To cite from Wikipedia (downloaded 24 May 2020) 'Geschwind attended Harvard Medical School, intending to become a psychiatrist. His emphasis began to shift after studying neuroanatomy with Marcus Singer, at which time he began to develop an interest in aphasia and epilepsy. He graduated medical school in 1951. Geschwind continued his studies at London's National Hospital, Queen Square, as a Moseley Travelling Fellow from 1952 to 1953, then as a United States Public Health Service fellow from 1953 to 1955. He studied with Sir Charles Symonds who taught the importance of neurologic mechanisms to studying disorders.

In 1955, Geschwind became neurology chief resident at the Boston City Hospital and served under Derek Denny-Brown. From 1956 to 1958 he was a research fellow studying muscle disease at the MIT Department of Biology. He joined the Neurology Department of the Boston Veterans Administration Hospital in 1958, where he met Fred Quadfasel, chief of neurology for the department. At this time, his clinical interest in aphasia developed into his lifelong study of the neurological basis of language and higher cognitive functions. Quadfasel encouraged Geschwind to study classic texts of neurology from the 19th and early twentieth century, exposing him to classic localisationist theory.

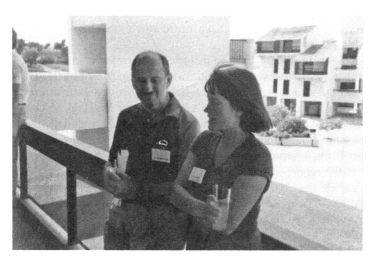

Figure 8.1 Norman Geschwind and Barbara at a meeting in Greece in 1984: Norman died about two months later.

So that was my first day in the new job in an area I would remain in for the rest of my career. I think any reader would have to agree it was pretty interesting, and I'm not surprised I fell in love with brain injury rehabilitation. I really enjoy the mixture of normality and abnormality seen in survivors of brain injury and the chance it offers to solve problems. The woman with apraxia was fascinating and probably did have a disconnection syndrome. I never wrote her up but did write up Derek and many other patients I saw at Rivermead.

In my case studies book, most of the patients are from RRC (Wilson 1999). Incidentally, this book won a book of the year award from the British Psychological Society in 2004. This may sound a long time after publication but the BPS has to wait for reviews to come in.

At RRC I worked closely with the other therapists who taught me a great deal. I wrote papers with some of them. Many patients presented clinical puzzles and after a while Alan Baddeley came to see some of them which led to a fruitful working relationship for a number of years. RRC was an NHS facility taking approximately one-third of patients from the Oxford district, one-third from the Oxfordshire region and one-third from the rest of the country. This was in the days before Margaret Thatcher and her government changed our lives to a more market economy (and changed the NHS for the worse): we had the principle of free referral which meant anyone could be referred for free to any NHS facility anywhere in the United Kingdom. We also had three social workers at RRC – three! – all of whom did a valuable job. I have not seen a social worker in day centres for people with brain injury in years, although I have heard there may be some in acute centres.

An amusing story I'd like to include here is when I was asked to see a woman with suspected dementia who was married to a lord. I saw her and did an assessment. In fact, her dementia was quite advanced. I said I would write the report and arrange for my assistant psychologist to see her at home to help with certain things. As they left, the husband said 'What about the erm …'. I thought he wanted a copy of the report I was to write and said that I would send him a copy. He said it wasn't the report, it was the bill! I laughed and said, 'Sorry, Lord … you are on the NHS today'. I told him I did not see private patients, his wife was being tested with the same tests and in the same room as everyone referred to me so he would not be charged. He then asked if I liked wine. I did not want any payment as my salary was paid by the health authority but I did not want to appear boorish so I said I did like wine. After several days a crate of wonderful claret was delivered to me! I think it was a brand supplied specially to the House of Lords.

Needless to say, Mick and I drank it. I felt guilty for a long time as I felt it violated my principle of not expecting patients to pay.

To finish this chapter I am going to quote directly from my journal to include some notes taken as it was written in the heat of battle as it were. The only things I have changed are the names of the people, patients and staff, involved in the interactions that took place in order to maintain anonymity. I wish to give readers a sense of the work ethic that existed within various professions involved in neuropsychological rehabilitation at Rivermead, and to experience vicariously what it was like working there with patients suffering from brain injury. So here it is straight from the horse's mouth.

Monday April 28th 1980

Weekend work – Saturday 1.5 hours on 2 reports (FG and OF), 2 hours on that paper for OD – I now have a rough draft - and 2.5 hours preparing for the IOP talk – I began a survey of the patients I've seen: 18 strokes, 5 tumours, 1 alcohol poisoning, 1 operation gone wrong, and 31 head injured 22 of whom were closed head injuries, 6 were fractures and 3 penetrating wounds. Also did ages on PTS (most between 16–25) as one would expect) + 2 gunshots, 2 industrial, 2 fights + 25 RTAs. Of the RTAs 9 were car drivers, 7 were pedestrians, 7 were motor cyclists + 2 were passengers. I found it all quite absorbing. Also on Sat morning B. Yule sent my copy of the Croom Helm book 'Behaviour Mod for the Mentally Handicapped.' It's actually quite a nice book although I couldn't bear reading my chapter and a half. It refers to notes about contributors where I'm working now and where I formerly worked. On Sunday I spent 4 hours preparing the handout and references for this talk ready for Pat to type (I meant to hand them in today but I literally did not have a spare minute to get them out of my bag and take over to her). Then I got on with my survey for a couple of hours– looked at V.I.Q.s, P.I.Qs, memory probs, reading probs, visuo-spatial probs and language probs. 90 % have memory probs, something like 50% have V-S+ perceptual probs and almost 50% have speech and/or lang probs and 39% reading probs. Finally spent an hour reading 'Techniques for efficient remembering', preparing for our memory group tomorrow (i.e. today). Arrived 8.50 today – had to sort out driving assessment and pts first. V did 4 people today, Eileen as a young normal, Bob as an old normal and 2 outside young normals this p.m. (Bob and Eileen we can do the IQ tests on another time). From 9.20–10.30 J and I saw DT first (v. confused and unmotivated. We don't know whether depressed or just can't understand I'm going to see him tomorrow and try some signs), and OY second. CJ came to watch O as she is going to give him extra sessions – she was also surprised at how low a level he is. After coffee I saw EV – she is very handicapped with her memory and visual perception problems. Then at 12 I dashed over to physio to see if I could change the beginning part of my film – arranged to do that this p.m. Also spoke to UO who is joining our memory group (that's useful as she can cope the days we are not available – arranged to see her with Mrs. J at 2 to explain what we are doing. Had a phone call from FD asking if she could come and see OV on Thurs. I said I'd ask the others and phone back. Then had to arrange with Helen V about the first driving assessment this afternoon. (I was tied up with the groups so asked if she'd do some of my testing) – gathered all the material together then went over all the paper and pencil tests with her (I didn't think she'd cope with the reaction time and pursuit rotor tests). By then it was one – had lunch - then dashed back to physio with the video film. D and T were not ready so I dashed back to OT – borrowed their blackboard for the memory group – took it over to my room – (2 trips) – wrote the first verse of "The Eagle" on the blackboard for one of the exercises – back to physio – added a piece of film of LR in place of the uninformative piece about O – back to Radley – 2.10 by then – quick discussion with U O and CJ. Patients arrived at 2.20. O – (star pupi), E (second best), G (not too bad) and C (weakest) – but in a reasonable mood. We taped most of the session (but I haven't heard it through yet). We began with 2 goes of Kim's Game then 'Mrs Brown went to town'. Both went down well. After that did the poem on blackboard The Eagle with me rubbing out a word at a time. We ended up with Pursuit Rotor, 1 minute each – but that was v. difficult for all of them except O. Didn't finish until 3.25. After tea Dr. U phoned (I'd asked S to phone back to F D about a 70 year old aphasic lady and F was making enquiries about sign language. Anyway, I said I'd ask CJ to bring it up at admissions meeting and we'd ring her back. From 3.45 to 5 I was tied up with the driving. The first young man and I managed to work out the choice of R.T. equipment - if we leave the top part off (with all the wires showing) and balance it on a cupboard box, it works more often than not. After 5 I cleared my room (which was in a bad way) discussed the group with C (we felt quite happy about it) and DT with Helen (he's very moody). Helen also loaned me her Speech Therapy Bulletin with an article in it saying speech therapists and psychologists are not cooperating enough. I think the 3 of us ought to reply saying how things are at RRC.

9 The disaster in the USA – 9/11 and memories of earlier times when we visited New York

Many people will remember where they were when the terrible terrorist attack in the USA in September 2001 occurred. I was at a brain injury meeting in Lincoln, England. It was the afternoon of 9 September when a woman I did not know, an attendee at the conference, asked me at the tea break, if I had heard what had happened in the USA. I had not heard and she said I should watch the television. I dashed back to my hotel room and watched with horror the destruction of the Twin Towers. I could not believe what I was seeing! It was only a year since Sarah died and our son, Matthew was in the USA in Manhattan where the terrorist attack occurred. I thought that if anything had happened to Matthew I could not go through it all again. I tried phoning him but the phone lines were dead. I phoned Mick who was also watching the news aghast and in disbelief. I asked if men had caused this. 'Of course it was!', he said. Part of me was hoping it was an accident and not a terrorist attack. I gave Mick two other phone numbers to try for Matthew who was staying with an ex-girlfriend in Manhattan. I returned to the conference where everybody was open mouthed and disbelieving.

I phoned Mick again that evening, and he had managed to speak to Matthew who was OK and had been in a different part of Manhattan when the disaster occurred. His girlfriend, though, had known one of the 343 firemen who had been killed while attempting to rescue people. Matt was able to get home a few days later.

We were still fragile from the loss of Sarah. Shortly after her death a year or so earlier we had visited Matt in the States as he was about to return to Philadelphia to continue his freelance photography. At that time we met up in New York where we had an emotional and tearful reunion. Soon after our arrival when I was jetlagged and still early on in grief, a group of Matt's friends took us to dinner at Bar 9. One of the girls had a call from a friend of hers who was in a car crash; we were told the car crash victim was screaming from the car and, apparently, I said that was a good thing as it showed she wasn't unconscious. I think I would have been more sympathetic if Sarah had not recently died. During the meal at Bar 9 I started to yawn, a wealthy young man at the dinner and known to be addicted to cocaine, leaned over and said 'Dr Wilson, can I offer you some cocaine'? I was very polite and replied. 'No thank you very much, I think I just need to head back to the hotel for an early night.' Matt said he and his friends laughed for a long time over that story.

We later drove to Lake Mohonk in upstate New York and stayed in a lovely old hotel, Mohonk Mountain Lodge, for two nights. This beautiful place is in the Shawangunk Ridge, Sky Top Mountain, close to the town of New Paltz. We even swam in the stunning lake which was bitterly cold despite the weather being sunny and warm. Lovely as this was we were still deep in grief.

We went to New York city several years after 9/11 with Francesca, our second granddaughter for her fifteenth birthday. Like her older sister, Rosie, Francesca was able to choose anywhere in the world to go for this birthday and, lockdown and coronavirus permitting, the two grandsons in Chile will also get to choose a special holiday when they reach 15. Well, Francesca chose to go to New York which Mick and I were happy about. We flew out from London and took a bus from the airport into the city. It was evening when we arrived and we could see the lights of the city as we neared our destination. New York never fails to impress. We did all the touristy things including the Empire State building, a Cole Porter show on Broadway and, one of the things Mick and I really like, a Sunday morning visit to Harlem to hear a gospel choir sing at a church service. While there, during the service, the maître d asked if anyone was there celebrating a special occasion. Francesca spoke up and said she was there for her fifteenth birthday. She was invited to the front and the choir sang a special song for her.

Of course, we had to visit Ground Zero, the spot where the World Trade Centre once stood. We were quiet remembering the terrible events of 9/11 and then went into the church nearest to Ground Zero partly because it seemed the right thing to do, even for non-believers like us and partly because it was a calm place to sit and reflect on the events that had happened to our family and to all those families affected by the disaster. This piece is taken from the website of the church (downloaded from http s://www.trinitywallstreet.org 27 May 2020).

After the attacks of September 11, 2001, St. Paul's Chapel, which sits directly across the street from the World Trade Center site, suffered no physical damage. On September 12, Lyndon Harris, then a priest on the clergy staff at Trinity and St. Paul's, arrived at

St. Paul's Chapel expecting major damage. He was amazed to find
that the church was without even a pane of glass broken. The
exterior of St Paul's and its churchyard were covered in debris.
After engineers inspected the building and pronounced it sound,
clean up began. As recovery work started at the World Trade
Center site, hundreds of rescue workers came to Lower Manhattan
to search for survivors and begin sorting through the ruins. Slowly
at first, rescue workers, police, and firefighters stopped by the
chapel to rest and wash up. Because long, exhausting shifts prevented many workers from going home, the chapel opened its
doors so that they could rest. Shortly after, an outdoor grill was
fired up, and volunteers began to serve food to hungry rescue and
recovery workers. Volunteers from Seamen's Church Institute
arrived on September 15 with food, clothing, and other supplies.
Labor of Love, an Episcopal relief ministry based in Asheville,
North Carolina, arrived on September 21. The volunteers were all
experienced in disaster relief and skilled in offering support and
guidance during a crisis. During all hours of the day and night,
rescue and recovery workers staggered through the gates of the
chapel. Hungry and weary, weighed down with gear, wearing boots
half-melted from the fiery ash, they fell into St. Paul's open embrace.
After working gruelling 12–18 hour shifts at Ground Zero, rescue
and recovery workers knew that St Paul's was a place they could rest
for a few hours before returning to the pit.

In the first three months after September 11, more than 3,000
workers passed through the chapel's gates. Police officers, Port
Authority workers, firefighters, National Guardsmen, construction
and sanitation crews, engineers and technicians found their way to
St. Paul's. The recovery workers were changed by what they
volunteered to do at Ground Zero, but they also were changed by
the ministry offered to them by St. Paul's and its volunteers.

I end this chapter with a quotation from the first memoirs book
about our feelings at the time.

> We thought out hearts were broken when we lost our firstborn child.
> Our hearts have healed, or at least the open wound has become a
> scar. We cry very readily. The disaster in the United States on Sep-
> tember 11th affected almost all the world, but we felt particularly
> affected as we knew how parents losing adult children would feel;
> particularly those who did not have a body to bury. Yet we felt their
> situation was worse than ours, for men had caused the deaths of the

people in New York, Washington and Pennsylvania. Sarah chose her white water rafting trip and was not the victim of brutality or terror. At times her death seems inevitable, at times we cannot really believe she is dead. We can laugh, enjoy ourselves, work, play, sleep, eat, despite this wound. The first year is hard, but as all bereaved parents say, 'You learn to live with it.' This is a cliché but it is also true. Sarah, we miss you, we love you, we will never forget you. You were our joy, our treasure, our precious gift and we will try to live our lives better because of you. (Wilson & Wilson 2004, p. 112)

10 Links with Chile

In the earlier memoirs book, I describe how Matt met Andrea. I also told the story about Pinochet and how I became involved with an evaluation of the Chilean dictator's so-called dementia. Here I will say more about my links with Chile, which I visit at least once a year (or did until the current coronavirus pandemic took control of our lives). As I write this on 29 May 2020, the British lockdown has been in place for over nine weeks. Although it looks as though the pandemic is easing a little here in Britain we still fear the infection rate might increase. There is also much anger about Dominic Cummings, chief adviser to the prime minister, Boris Johnson, but I shall refer to these matters more fully in a later chapter.

Back to my links with Chile. My first trip there was in 2002 just after Matt told me about the wonderful Chilean girl, Andrea, he had met in Brighton. I said that as I had to go to Chile soon, Matt could come with me and meet up with Andrea again. I was giving a talk at a conference in Santiago de Chile on that occasion and I have been there several times since. Santiago, like many other places in Chile has some wonderful restaurants. With such a long coastline, it is almost bound to have good fish and seafood. To give one an idea of the length of the country, I once read that if Chile were transferred to Europe it would stretch from Norway to Tunisia. Of course it is extremely thin being bounded by the Andes and the sea for most of its length. I love the seafood and fish there, one of my favourite dishes being ceviche and, in South America, I regularly choose this if it is on the menu. The best ceviche I have ever had was in Santiago at a good fish restaurant called Aqui Esta Coco. We also like the restaurants in Santa Cruz where Matt, Andrea, Sammy and Max live. One is Viu Manent, a winery with a good restaurant attached, where we often go for lunch as we can walk there from Matt's house. We also like the Peruvian restaurant in that town, and Casa Colchuaga, which is Mick's favourite, with its astonishing variety of dishes. Just out of town and set in the middle of a beautiful winery is Vic where the meat is cooked in open fires and accompanied by delicious red wines from the vineyard where we sometimes go for special occasions. Lapostolle, the winery where Andrea works, has a good restaurant too and, if one wants to splash out, their casitas (little houses) set in the foothills of the mountains, are wonderful places to stay. The countryside is stunning, the pool lovely and the little houses well equipped.

There are lots of tarantulas in Chile and sometimes, one of my grandsons will find one in the garden for me to hold and admire. They are not poisonous and are rather beautiful. I get cross with people who don't like spiders or snakes. Both creatures, to me, have their own beauty and, like all of us, are just trying to get through life in the best way possible. I am sometimes seen as a strange gringo lady who likes tarantulas! But they really are harmless.

In the first book, I described Matt and Andrea's wedding in a winery in Santiago which was conducted half in Spanish and half in English. Anna, Rosie and Francesca were there too and we had a holiday afterwards. For a while we thought the wedding might have to be cancelled as it was planned for the same time as a big exposition of leaders of countries from the Pacific Rim were meeting there and many hotels were fully booked with government officials and leaders, including George W. Bush from the USA.

For the days of the actual wedding, we managed to book two rooms at the Sheraton Hotel in Santiago. A very pleasant hotel that we have since stayed at several times. The security at the hotel was very strict because a number of important people were staying there. I remember that on one occasion I was waiting for the lift to take me to my room when a member of staff told me I could not take the next lift. I asked why not and he said 'Because Korean First Lady coming'. I really did not see why I could not travel in the same lift as the Korean first lady. George W. Bush, then president of the United States was at the same meeting, although not in the same hotel. We learned that he had his armed bodyguards with him and that guns were not permitted in a certain meeting which he was attending. We read in the press that there was a confrontation between Bush's bodyguards and the Chilean security, which consisted of many soldiers. Bush's guards had to give way and were prevented from entering the actual meeting room. For a moment a picture was captured in some of the press showing President Bush helplessly trying to get to his own guards but not being able to break through the line of Chilean soldiers. The Chileans loved seeing that in their newspapers and regarded their soldiers as heroes for a moment or two! When in Chile do as the Chileans do.

On another occasion we were staying at the same hotel in Santiago with Matt who had a separate room. We had taken a taxi to go somewhere and Matt had left a borrowed camera in the taxi! He was upset, we told the reception desk who asked if we had booked the taxi through the hotel. We had and they said not to worry, they would trace the taxi and the camera would be returned. This happened much to our relief and confirmed our views that the Sheraton was a good place to stay.

After the wedding Mick, Anna, Rosie, Francesca and I went on a cruise, not the one departing from the very south in Punta Arenas where we had hoped to see elephant seals (as this was fully booked by the people at the big meeting). Instead we went on another cruise departing from Puerto Montt at the southern end of the Chilean Central Valley. This was, to be honest, a little boring for us all as we spent a week on the cruise with very few trips ashore. We did get to see the San Rafael Glacier, though which was impressive. This glacier, which can be seen for miles because if its size and steep descent, flows into a glacial saltwater lake. It is also the nearest glacier to the equator. We travelled to it from the cruise ship in Zodiac boats.

I have travelled fairly extensively in Chile, sometimes with Mick, sometimes with Matthew and sometimes with others. One of our favourite places is Easter Island or Rapa Nui to give it its native title. Matthew and I first went there on our second trip to Chile in 2003. We flew from Santiago, a five hour trip over the Pacific Ocean. In fact, it is only possible to fly to Rapa Nui from Santiago de Chile or from Tahiti. We had only two days there so booked two trips to see the famous moai statues, which are absolutely stunning. This is what Wikipedia has to say (downloaded 30 May 2020):

> **Easter Island** *(Rapa Nui: Rapa Nui, Spanish: Isla de Pascua) is an island and special territory of Chile in the southeastern Pacific Ocean, at the southeastern most point of the Polynesian Triangle in Oceania. Easter Island is most famous for its nearly 1,000 extant monumental statues, called moai, created by the early Rapa Nui people. In 1995, UNESCO named Easter Island a World Heritage Site, with much of the island protected within Rapa Nui National Park.*
>
> *It is believed that Easter Island's Polynesian inhabitants arrived on Easter Island sometime near 1200 AD. They created a thriving and industrious culture, as evidenced by the island's numerous enormous stone moai and other artifacts. However, land clearing for cultivation and the introduction of the Polynesian rat led to gradual deforestation. By the time of European arrival in 1722, the island's population was estimated to be 2,000–3,000. European diseases, Peruvian slave raiding expeditions in the 1860s, and emigration to*

other islands, e.g. Tahiti, further depleted the population, reducing it to a low of 111 native inhabitants in 1877.

Chile annexed Easter Island in 1888. In 1966, the Rapa Nui were granted Chilean citizenship. In 2007 the island gained the constitutional status of "special territory" (Spanish: territorio especial). The 2017 Chilean census registered 7,750 people on the island, of whom 3,512 (45%) considered themselves Rapa Nui. Easter Island is one of the most remote inhabited islands in the world.

In fact Mick and I have been to *the* remotest inhabited island which is Tristan Da Cunha in the South Atlantic but that is another story.

During this first trip to Rapa Nui, Matt was still collecting football shirts and has a collection of over 150 (the most expensive of which Mick and I bought him when we were in Kyoto). He wanted one from Rapa Nui and we saw a local football game while on a walk near the hotel. Matt talked to the people to ask if we could buy one of their shirts (there were none for sale in the shops). They said, no so it looked as if we were unsuccessful and we gave up. However, later that evening while we were asleep in the hotel room, one of the hotel staff woke us up to say there were some local people there with a football shirt they said we wanted! We got up, met the people and paid for the football shirt, so Matt did manage to buy one after all. This may not seem much to you, the reader, but to actually own a shirt from a football team based on Easter Island is we think a real treasure. It may be unique!

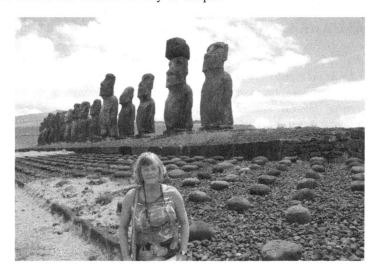

Figure 10.1 Some of the moais in Easter Island.

Several years later, we went to Rapa Nui again for New Year with the Chilean family. Mick was suitably impressed with the island and loved the huge and stunning moai, which do not face the sea but all look inland. The island is not manicured like Hawaii but rough and ready. There are horses everywhere and all the locals seem to ride. We learned of the history of the island, how all the trees were destroyed and the ritual of the strange bird men. There used to be a ceremony on the island in the form of an annual competition to collect the first sooty tern's egg of the season from a nearby tiny island. The young men would swim out collect the egg, then swim back to Rapa Nui and climb the sea cliff to a cliff top village. Christian missionaries stopped the ritual in the 1860s. The origin of the cult of the Bird Men is unclear as it is unknown whether the cult replaced the preceding moai-based religion or had co-existed with it. I remember being on the Cook Islands with Pauline Monro and listening to a history of the islands where the people are Maori. Legend has it that there were 12 tribes who set off across the sea, two tribes were lost and the rest settled in various places including Rapa Nui. Most of the settlers looked after the environment well but the ones who settled on Rapa Nui seemed to destroy their environment by cutting down all the trees to transport the moai. The drawings, statues and symbols of the bird men always show them as being very emaciated as if they were starving.

We have also visited the Atacama Desert in the north of the country, one of my favourite places in Chile. The scenery there has been compared to that of Mars, and it is very dramatic, it is one of the driest places on earth and certainly the driest nonpolar desert. Because of its high altitude, extremely limited cloud cover, dry air, lack of light pollution and radio interference from widely populated cities and towns, this desert is one of the best places in the world to conduct astronomical observations.

Most visitors to Chile seem to go on wine tours and Chile certainly has fantastic wine, indeed our daughter-in-law, Andrea Leon, was voted best winemaker in Chile in 2016; the only time a woman has won this prestigious award. Chile is the fifth largest wine producing country in the world. Another place worth visiting, if you ever go to this fascinating and beautiful country, is Pucon, almost 800 kilometres south of Santiago. Pucon is home to Villarrica, one of the most active volcanoes in Latin America. We were there with the Chilean family and went in two cars. The weather wasn't wonderful but we had a good time including a great day out at one of the thermal pools, of which there are many in Chile. The area is the land of the Mapuche, the indigenous people of this region and one of the peoples never conquered by the Spanish.

Another thing I like about South America is the Day of the Dead held to celebrate all those who have died. It is held on 1 November and, if we are in a South American Country we go to a cemetery to remember Sarah and celebrate her life. The year she died, a colleague, Fergus Gracey, was travelling in South America and left flowers for Sarah on the Day of the Dead. In 2019 we were in Chile on 1 November so went to the local cemetery with Matthew. We bought flowers for Sarah at the gates of the cemetery and walked around. Typically, Chilean cemeteries are colourful and not at all sad like British cemeteries. People go with their families, dress up and have picnics on this particular day. There is a section for children which is moving and one can read the stories of how the children died. I was obviously filled with sorrow (see the photo on page XXX) and did not know where to leave the flowers we had brought as most people left theirs at the graves of the person who had departed. Then we spotted a rather barren place for old people who had died. There were hardly any flowers there so, having decided that Sarah would approve of her flowers being left for the abandoned old people, we left them there. On leaving the cemetery, we saw a man begging so I gave him some money in memory of our daughter.

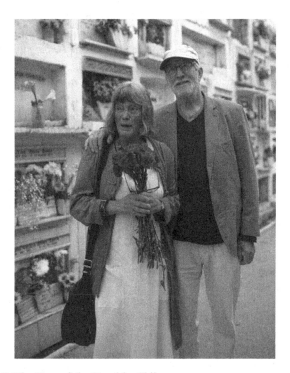

Figure 10.2 The Day of the Dead in Chile.

Not only is Chile famous for the Andes, its wine, its thermal pools and the Day of the Dead, it is one of the world's hotspots for earthquakes. Many will remember the terrible earthquake in Haiti in 2010 with the loss of many lives. This was a magnitude of 7.00 on the Richter scale. Few, however, will remember that in February of the same year an even larger earthquake struck Chile with a magnitude of 8.8! Fewer lives were lost in Chile partly because of the less dense population and partly because of stronger buildings. Nevertheless, it was a terrible experience for the Chileans even though they are used to earthquakes. Of all the major earthquakes in the world since 1500, one-third have occurred in Chile. When the very large one started in 2010, my daughter-in-law who has experienced several earthquakes woke up and thought at first it was a tremor, my son was not sure, then Andrea shouted, 'It's the real thing!' and it was indeed.

She told Matt to get Sammy, then 4 years old, and she would get Max, who was not quite 2 years old. They went for the children who were in bed and Sammy asked why his father was shaking the bed.

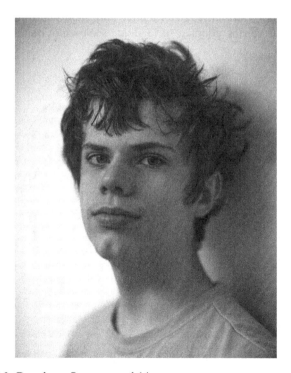

Figure 10.3 Grandson, Sammy, aged 14 years.

Matt said the concrete floor was rolling in waves! They all escaped harm but lost £5,000 worth of smashed furniture, glass and wine bottles in their house. The next time I saw the boys they were playing earthquakes with their toy trucks. I said I had never been in an earthquake and they explained, in a matter of fact way, what happened in theirs. The closest Mick and I ever came to an earthquake, was one morning while staying at a hotel next to the airport in Santiago just before flying home, the bed shook and I realised we had experienced a tremor. Mick pointed out that 'No' we had not been making love!

In addition to visiting family, I have been to Chile several times for work, my closest colleague being Christian Salas who works at Diego Portales University. Christian worked for several years in the United Kingdom where I first met him. I have given three lectures at Diego Portales University. Indeed, Christian Salas is, perhaps, the only person in Chile to be engaged in the kind of rehabilitation I recognise. Although he describes himself as a psychoanalytical psychotherapist (which I most certainly am not), his main interest is to understand the emotional and personality changes after brain injury and how psychoanalytic tools can be adapted to facilitate socio-emotional adjustment

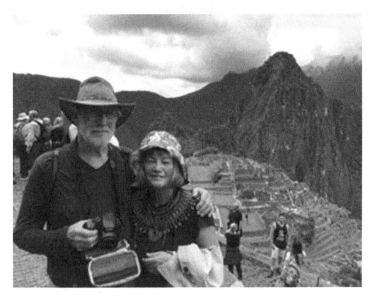

Figure 10.4 We climbed Macchu Pichu in 2019: Mick, aged 84 was considered the hero of the group because he was the oldest member. I am a mere 77 years.

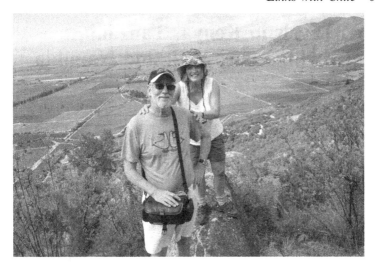

Figure 10.5 Mick and Barbara in one of the Chilean vineyards.

and well-being. This is not so different from us at the Oliver Zangwill Centre helping with the emotional and identity difficulties faced by survivors of brain injury. I feel a loyalty to Chile which, although not perfect, is certainly beautiful and perhaps the least corrupt of the South American countries. They are going through hell now though with the coronavirus. Matt says most people won't socially distance and won't wear masks.

11 Travels in Kenya, Tanzania, Madagascar, Mali and Namibia

My marriage, babies, evening classes, university days as a mature student and my introduction to brain injury rehabilitation have been covered in the previous book. Interspersed with these 'adventures', I have remained a keen and serious traveller both for work and pleasure. In this chapter, I describe some of the exciting places I have visited for pleasure, sometimes alone and sometimes with members of my family. Up until April 2020, I have stayed in over 100 independent countries, and been on 23 safaris; 20 in Africa and 3 in India.

For those of you who have read the earlier book you will know that our favourite holidays, that is for Mick and me, are safaris. These offer an adventure experienced in a landscape as near to wilderness as you are likely to get in the modern world. As others have noted, there is a special feeling when you enter a wilderness, which is missing from our daily lives in modern times. Mick has always argued that one needs to read Wordsworth's poetry to remind oneself of those feelings experienced only in the wilderness that are missing now in modern life in the UK but were still there, in Britain, at the beginning of the nineteenth century. As Wordsworth describes it, the experience one gets is 'Felt in the blood, and felt along the heart.' In the first book I tried to recreate those feelings when I described our sightings of lions, a martial eagle and a pack of wild dogs.

The very first safari I went on was in South Africa in 1995. I would not go to South Africa during the apartheid era and Mick and I protested about the regime, refusing to buy South African goods and, in Mick's case, after receiving advice from the African National Congress, refusing to sell tests to the white South African government. In 1995 though, after the regime ended, I accepted an invitation to speak in Johannesburg, and stayed with Victor Nell and his wife, Myrna. They later moved to the UK where Victor died in 2007. After the lecture, I went on a cheap safari to Skukuza Lodge in the Kruger National Park.

I stayed in a hostel, travelled in a vehicle with many others, mostly back-packers but managed to enjoy myself and see a number of animals.

A better experience, and accompanied by Mick and our oldest grand-daughter, Rosie, was in Kenya in 1996 or thereabouts. It came about because of Mick's youngest sister, Carol, who is a little younger than me and who was so helpful when Sarah died. At the time, Carol was married to Peter, who sadly died of emphysema two years ago. Peter, a journalist, was working in Nairobi. Kenya, for one of the two national Kenyan newspapers. Carol divided her time between the UK and Nairobi. One day, she was talking to Rosie and said she should persuade her grand-parents to take her to Kenya. Of course, we did. We organised a trip, including a safari, with a rather cheap company (I would not use again) which included a few days in Zanzibar in Tanzania. We were going to Mombasa, in Kenya, after the safari but heard reports of riots there so chose Zanzibar instead. After an overnight flight and a change of planes we landed in Nairobi and Peter's driver, Mohammed, met us to take us to Carol and Peter's very pleasant house. The maid was called Esther and she really took a shine to Rosie. Carol did not like having a maid as this was not usual in the UK for people like us but it was expected in Kenya and offered employment to local people. Carol told me that when she first went to Nairobi and met Esther, she would try to help in the kitchen but as Carol was peeling vegetables or whatever, a pair of black hands would appear and try to take over so, eventually, Carol gave up.

After we had refreshed ourselves and had a sleep, Peter took us out in his land rover to a nearby game park to see some animals. Rosie was allowed to sit on the roof of the vehicle with us and she could hardly believe this was permitted. I went to this same park many years later with my friend and colleague, Shai Betteridge, after a trip to Rwanda to search for gorillas. The gorilla trek was probably the best safari I have ever had. We were so close to the wonderful mountain gorillas that I fell in love with the first male silverback I encountered. Back to our first safari in Kenya: before we left for the six-day trip, Esther took Rosie to meet her friends and they both had a good time.

A few days later, we went to meet our group and set off for the first camp, Samburu. There was a mother and her 11-year-old son, Alex, in the same vehicle as us. Rosie and Alex became good friends and were inseparable during our holiday. Samburu was fascinating, we were entertained by the Samburu dancers who jumped high into the air. I think little 9-year-old Rosie was rather frightened of them but they were truly wonderful. Another thing about that camp was the naughty monkeys who tried to steal our breakfast things. The staff were cross and discouraged the monkeys but the visitors loved them. There was a

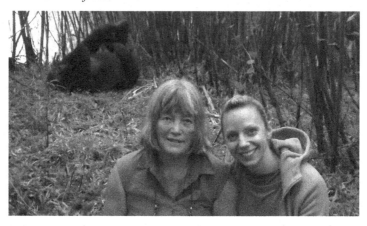

Figure 11.1 Barbara and Shai with gorilla in background: trekking in Rwanda.

huge crocodile at the camp, it was fed every evening and the visitors sat in rows while the huge crocodile lumbered up from the river along the grass for its nightly lump of meat. The birds there were stunning, carmine bee eaters, lilac crested rollers, magnificent starlings and others. We also saw lions, elephant and buffalo. These are three of the big five, the other two being rhinoceros and leopard. We have seen the big five many times on our safaris but not in Kenya. Rhinos are heavily poached there. Our best rhino viewing has always been in South Africa where it is easier to see leopards too. In Kenya, I learned about the little five which are the lion ant, the elephant shrew, the buffalo weaver, the leopard tortoise and the rhinoceros beetle. Since that first safari, I have seen four of the little five but never an elephant shrew (except on television).

From Samburu we travelled to Lake Navasha, another beautiful spot. We were sitting having Sunday lunch there when who should come across the grass but Carol and Peter! They had driven from Nairobi to meet us for lunch and a walk around the lake. Our last camp was at the Masai Mara where we were fortunate enough to see the great migration of the wildebeest. Thousands of them thundered past. The van would drive slowly, stop and then continue through this seething mass of creatures. On one of the journeys we had stopped at a market and bought an old Masai mask to go with our small collection of African sculptures. Later we met a very old Masai woman and showed her the mask we had bought. She reverently touched the mask in several places saying 'Masai, Masai, Masai' each time.

The number of animals we saw on the plains was extraordinary and it was the beginning of our love of safaris. As Mick often says, they are the best holidays: you are in real wilderness but stay in luxurious lodges and never know what the day is going to bring. The van broke down on one of the journeys and we had to pile out while the driver fixed it. Rosie said 'Where are the sellers?' I realised that everywhere we had been until that point, we had been surrounded by people selling us things but this was an unscheduled stop so there were no people encouraging us to buy.

Several local people asked us how we pronounced the name of their country. We said Kenya (with a short 'e'). This was approved of as they did not like 'Keenya' which is how the British settlers there pronounced the name. Of course, I remembered the Mau Mau who fought for Kenyan independence when I was a child. I always supported those movements for independence anyway, although not always the methods used. We talked to other people in the camps and said we were going on to Zanzibar (which belonged to Tanzania) afterwards. Some asked if we had any problems getting our visas for Tanzania. We had not known that we needed visas for that country so had done nothing. We were advised we needed to sort these out before leaving for Zanzibar so phoned Peter in Nairobi and he said we could get the visas there before leaving the country.

After the safari, Mohammed met us in Nairobi with his beautifully kept vehicle and plush upholstered seats which was appreciated after the dilapidated van we had been travelling in. He also took us, the following day, to the Tanzanian embassy where we obtained our visas. This took several hours and cost us more than we expected but we were now able to enter the country.

We made our goodbyes, promising to return and tipped all the staff. We learned that Esther was saving up for a corrugated iron roof for her house in her village and that our tip was going towards that. We did return one year later, without Rosie and had another safari as well as a trip to Mount Kenya. Soon after this, Peter had to leave Nairobi as he had problems with the then prime minister Daniel Moi. Peter had to be very careful what his paper said about Moi. No jokes or cartoons were allowed. If Moi was mentioned, some official had to check the acceptance of the piece. Moi wanted Peter to employ people of a particular tribe but Peter said he would employ the best people no matter what the tribe. He stuck to his guns but problems became worse until Peter felt he had no choice but to leave the country and return to the UK.

Back to our trip. We arrived by air in Zanzibar and were driven to our hotel along the coast. One trip we took while there was to an old

Arab castle which had an ancient toilet arrangement that intrigued me. People sat on a stone wall and their urine and faeces dropped into the sea! We also saw some huge land tortoises which were very impressive. The capital of Zanzibar is Stonetown and we went there twice. I bought a beautiful old silver necklace for a reasonable price and kept it for two years until it was stolen in Cuba. More about the Cuba trip in a later chapter.

We never returned to Zanzibar but we did go back to Tanzania with Anna, Rosie and Francesca when Francesca was 9 years old. As Rosie had gone on her first safari when she was 9 years old we thought Francesca should also go on her first safari at the same age. The two boys in Chile also went but they were a little older (11 and 12 years) and we took them, not to Tanzania or Kenya but to South Africa.

Francesca's safari happened immediately after Christmas. We flew first to Dar Es Salaam, the largest town in Tanzania and immediately were taken by a small private plane with just enough seats for the five of us and the pilot, to Arusha where we spent the night. The pilot said one person could sit in front with him so we let Francesca sit there as it was her special holiday. As soon as the plane took off though, Francesca vomited and the pilot, so proud of his new plane, was horrified. She vomited several times more in the cockpit with Anna trying to

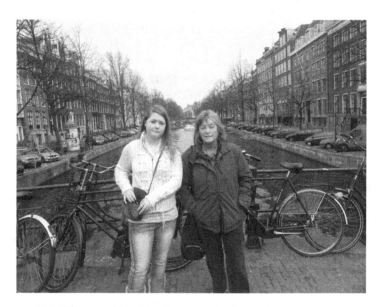

Figure 11.2 With granddaughter Francesca in Amsterdam.

clean up as best she could. For many years, Francesca suffered from air sickness. We spent a pleasant enough evening in Arusha before going on yet another small plane to Klein's Camp, a private game reserve in the Serengeti National Park.

We landed in a large airfield, hardly distinguishable from other fields in the area, surrounded by giraffe and zebra. It was quite magical. A guide from the camp had set up a table with drinks and snacks to welcome us, and the plane drove right up to the table before stopping. He told us there had just been a lion kill on the way to the lodge and asked if we would like to go there first before driving to the lodge for our lunch! We did this, feeling Francesca was lucky to have such a good start to her safari. We all loved Klein's Camp and it remains one of our favourite safaris. I think I am an expert in them now having visited so many in different parts of Africa.

On New Year's Eve we were driven to Ngorongoro crater which we had heard was one of the best places for a safari. It wasn't the best for

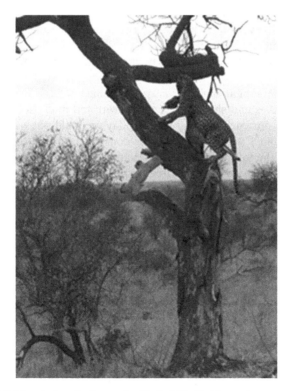

Figure 11.3 My photo of a leopard with its kill climbing a tree.

us though as there were very few animals and too many vehicles all chasing one or two or a few creatures. We saw far fewer animals than we had in Kenya or in Klein's Camp. What was magnificent though in Ngorongoro was the lodge we stayed in. It had chandeliers in the toilets! Between us we had two rooms and each had its own butler! The most special moment for me was the celebration on New Year's Eve. We were asked to walk from our rooms to the dining room for the special dinner. We walked through a long line of Masai warriors on either side of the path. Each carried a lighted torch making a tunnel for us to walk through. Francesca, a little girl walked through this line of warriors and torches as if it were a perfectly normal thing to do but, for me, the sight was breathtaking.

One of the most interesting African countries I have visited is Madagascar. I went there alone and it was my last safari before Sarah died in Peru in May 2000. Her death is covered in the previous book but I say more about it and how we are 20 years later in Chapter 15. I started travelling alone in the 1990s as Mick had an arthritic knee and could barely walk. This was eventually replaced and ever since Mick has been able to walk without any problems and no pain.

I wanted to go to Madagascar because of the unusual wildlife there and booked a 17-day trip with Explore Worldwide. We flew to Antananarivo, the capital of Madagascar. It rained for the first few days and our clothes and shoes were covered with red mud. Because of the weather and our back packing type holiday we could not wash and dry things. I found I was fed up with the constant rain and dirty clothes. Once out in the forest, I needed to pee and sought permission from our guide, Belinda, to go behind a tree. Either I went too far or the group moved but I lost them. I wandered around for a while in a mild state of panic and then found another group. I explained to the guide what had happened and with no trouble at all, he led me to my own group. I have always had a poor sense of direction. Even though we were in a forest then, much of Madagascar is seriously deforested as the people cut down the trees for charcoal. We were shocked at the amount of deforestation we saw around us.

Things improved after that when we moved further south. We saw a selection of most of the country's lemurs which are only found in Madagascar, and other creatures like tree frogs which were very colourful. I loved the Spiny Forest where almost all of the plants were prickly. We saw sifakas there, my favourite of the lemurs. Sifakas appear to dance as they bounce and leap along the ground. They were a constant source of wonder.

Even further south we went to a special area where there were many ring tailed lemurs. We were warned to keep our windows and doors closed at all times because the lemurs would get in and steal things. Of course, most of the tourists found this amusing. There was even a 'ring tailed lemur rehabilitation centre' there where the very naughty lemurs were captured and kept behind bars. I think they had bitten people and I believe they were not rehabilitated but always imprisoned.

On the road once while driving a long distance from one camp to another, we came across a nasty road accident. We stopped and there was a distressed woman holding an injured child and a baby. She wanted help but Belinda, the guide, said she was not allowed to take non-tourists in the van. We all rebelled and said she had to help so the local Malagasy woman and her two children came in the van with us and we went to the local hospital. It was a very basic place not like the hospitals in the UK but they took the woman and the children and said they would look after the little girl. We never found out what happened and I hope the injured child recovered. We continued our journey in a sombre mood. People seemed to like us driving through their country and often came to wave at us. We once saw a most beautiful garden full of lovely flowers. I asked the man who was obviously the owner of the garden (as well as the gardener) if I could take a photograph and he stood proudly by while I photographed him in his gorgeous garden. All in all the trip was worthwhile but there were problems as we seemed to divide into two factions with lots of quarrelling. This spilled over at the airport on the way home when a woman in our group (our faction) quarrelled over an airport trolley with a couple from the other faction! I tried to keep out of it.

One of my favourite trips was to Mali in north west Africa. I went there in 2001 because I wished to see Timbuktu. I mentioned Mali in the previous book but did not say much about the trip itself, only that Michael Palin was making a programme for the BBC at the time and I saw him once while in the toilets in Djenne. Once again, I travelled with Explore Worldwide and met the group I was with at London Heathrow. We flew to Paris first and then a long flight to Conakry in Guinea before the final flight to Bamako, the capital of Mali where we spent a pleasant two days at a decent hotel. I liked Bamako and learned that the famous English footballer, Bobby Charlton had stayed there.

After Bamako we drove to Mopti a big market town and visited a large, noisy, colourful, African market. The highlight of the trip though was not Timbuktu, interesting as that was, but our six-day trip with the Dogon tribe. The Dogon people live in a region of south-central Mali known for its secluded villages which are built into high cliffs. UNESCO listed this as a World Heritage Site in 1989. We had a Dogon guide there, Dao, a beautiful tall man, dressed in traditional white robes. Once in Dogon country which is on the edge of the Bandiagara Escarpment which, in turn, is on the edge of the Sahara Desert, we saw no cars or vehicles of any kind. We stayed in different villages and really experienced tribal life. The chief of each village we visited came to meet us. The chief and Dao exchanged a long greeting which translated as something like (Chief) 'How are you?' (Dao) 'I am fine. How are you?' (Chief) I am fine. How is your wife?' (Dao) 'My wife is fine. How is your wife?' (Chief) 'My wife is fine. How are your children?' (Dao) 'My children are fine. How are your children?'

The Dogon tribe is famous for its carvings and on our first night, we were fortunate enough to see a masked dance. The masks are huge and beautiful and the dance we saw was mesmerising. Some villages had a school and some did not. If there was a school in the village we were invited to see it and listen to the children sing, which we found very moving. We were also asked to donate to the school. If the village did not have a school, the chief asked us, with Dao translating, if we would donate some money to help them build a school. We typically donated in the region of $10 (US) each.

There were 17 people in the group plus our British leader a young man with a good first aid kit. There was also an American nurse from San Francisco who was wealthy and had brought a large amount of money with her. At every village, the guide and the nurse set up a clinic and the local people came with their sicknesses and illnesses. If it was a burn or something our 'local clinical team' felt they could deal with, they helped. If it was more serious, the nurse gave the chief some money and asked the chief to get the sick person to a hospital as more serious treatment was required. I was impressed with these two and their quiet professionalism. One evening sitting around after dinner we asked who would be needed the most should we all be stuck in Mali. The nurse was top of the list, one of the men in the group was a dentist and one a mechanic, we felt they would both be useful. As a clinical neuropsychologist I came way down the list because, although there were survivors of brain injury in Mali, I specialised only in patients after the early medical stages.

After the wonderful Dogon trip, we went to Djenne which has the largest mud mosque in the world and is stunning. That is where I saw Michael Palin and the film crew from the BBC. We were shocked at the crates of alcohol including excellent wine that they had with them. We were managing on beer or very poor Malian wine. However, we all shared the same hostel, so there was some equality!

Our final stop was to be Timbuktu which required a three day boat journey down the river Niger. This was an interesting experience. Not only did we see beautiful women in stunning clothes and excited children, we were caught in a serious dust storm. We had to stay in our tents until the storm passed and our food was brought round to us. As some tents were in danger of being blown away, a few people were moved into different tents to make them heavier. I shared with a woman called Eily and we did not have to move but there was a married couple who did. The wife, originally from Scandinavia, was a large, heavy woman and she was asked to move into a tent with a much smaller woman to make it heavier. During the night we heard her husband call out, 'Greta, Greta'. His wife called back, 'Yes?' to which the husband shouted 'I love you, Greta'. We thought that was funny.

By the next day, the storm had passed and we continued to Timbuktu. That town is inhabited by the Tuareg tribe who also wear colourful costumes. Timbuktu is renowned for its doors and we were told that only certain families are allowed to make the doors and some have been making them for hundreds of years. In its heyday, the city was a centre for Islamic learning and had a famous library but nowadays Timbuktu is impoverished and the desert is encroaching.

It was finally time to leave Mali and set off home. First we went back to Bamako, stayed in a good hotel and spent a day by the swimming pool. Today, one cannot visit this wonderful country unless for essential travel. This is because in 2012 militants took over northern Mali following the collapse of neighbouring Libya. The Foreign Office currently warns against all travel in northern Mali north of Segou and against all but essential travel in the south of the country. They say that the provinces of Tombouctou, Kidal, Gao and Mopti are totally off limits due to the risk of kidnapping and terrorist attack.

The journey home was an adventure in itself. We departed from Bamako airport. Although we all joined the queue at the same time, people jumping the queue meant we were separated from one another and I was pushed further and further back. We were flying first to Paris with Air Afrique (an airline that no longer exists) and then to London with Air France. Only the ones at the front of the queue were given boarding cards from Paris to London. I missed out and this meant I could not take the plane I was meant to be on from Paris to London. I had to take a later plane. It was not a disaster but after such a long journey any delay is unwelcome. The worst part of the long journey from Bamako to Paris is that there were cockroaches on the plane! This is the one and only time in the hundreds of flights I have taken where I saw cockroaches on an aeroplane.

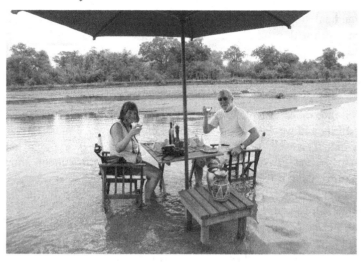

Figure 11.4 Having lunch in a river in Namibia. We did not see any crocodiles.

The final safari I mention in this chapter is one to Namibia that Mick and I took after Sarah died. This came about because I entered an online auction to bid for a trip to Namibia. I cannot remember how much I bid but I won. This isn't as wonderful as it sounds as we had to pay for our own flights to Windhoek, plus a night there as well as the holiday money we had bid. We did have a great time though and fell in love with Namibia even though we were not so impressed with the main safari park there, Etosha. We flew via South Africa to Windhoek and stayed a night there before joining our group. We were on a flying holiday so all the internal journeys were by air. At every camp we stayed, the staff sang a welcome to us, when we arrived, in their famous click language. That was special. Our favourite place was a wonderful camp called Sossusvlei which offered trips around special areas of sand dunes that themselves consisted of a territory so big that it is an obvious feature globally when viewed from space. The camp itself consisted of a few extremely well-constructed, permanent tents which could be described as lion and elephant proofed. There was no electricity in the camp but the manager and his wife explained that we had been supplied with special steam-controlled klaxon alarms that could be set off if anything disastrous were to take place in the night. We all laughed comfortably when they pointed out reassuringly that in 17 years no one had ever set off one of these alarms.

We finished that first night in the new camp with a twilight vigil as we watched many oryx that Namibia is known for. We then retired to our tents that could be safely zip locked from inside. As with all the previous camps, we had been warned to check our socks and shoes in the morning as scorpions had been known to settle into them after a night's foraging for prey. In fact that was all we had ever been told about scorpions so we were left in our ignorance regarding them as perhaps a single venomous species best to be avoided. Then at about 3.00 a.m. I was woken by a stifled scream from Mick, who leapt out of his bed, clutching his eye and shouting 'I've been stung!' I assumed it was a mosquito bite and was more concerned about the need to rise at 5.00 a.m for the safari. Mick would not let me return to sleep and said, 'Barbara, it is serious, I can smell a chemical'. I climbed out of bed and Mick raised his pillow. There was a small greyish wriggling scorpion there. 'Don't hurt it'! I cried. 'Rescue it'. 'Rescue it!' repeated Mick. 'I am going to kill it'. He hammered it with a book until it was dead. Now what was to be done? Mick was running round the bed saying he was going to die and I stood there helpless. Mick's eyes alighted on the klaxon and he said he was going to set it off so that the owners could come and rescue him. I suggested that this was perhaps a bit too dramatic, thinking about those 17 years during which it had never been sounded. What would the other campers think when they heard it? How frightened might they be! But Mick was determined, grabbed the alarm and set it off. We waited for a few minutes and nobody came. Mick, very impatient, said he was going to go and find help. I said that he shouldn't go outside as there could be lions around. Ignoring me, Mick set off to find help from the staff. I knew he hadn't been attacked as I could hear the klaxon getting fainter in the distance. We learned later that all the other tourists had woken up, pulled the covers over their faces and waited for the lions to attack. Mick continued to swing the alarm around in the dark, hoping to be rescued by knowledgeable camp leaders but no one came for ten or more minutes during which time the klaxon continued to ruin the dark and mysterious African night. What must the animals have thought? I waited anxiously in the tent and until, eventually six members of staff plus Mick, turned up in our tent. They had taken so long because their accommodation was at the other end of the camp and they had to get dressed. The manager asked what kind of scorpion it was and we showed him the poor dead little creature under the pillow. We were told that Mick wouldn't die and it wasn't a very venomous scorpion. The manager's wife, in charge of first aid, was at a loss at what to do. She asked me if she should give him antibiotics! I could not believe her. 'Antibiotics?' I queried. 'For a scorpion sting? No, certainly not'. She then said 'Well I don't know what to do, the nearest doctor is over two hours drive away'. Feeling cross at her incompetence, I said 'One of the other guests, Bob, is a medical doctor from Australia. I suggest you go and ask him to come'. Bob duly appeared, looked at the bite and did several checks. He said to put ice on it and it would go in two or three days. It would be no worse than a wasp sting. The manager had ice in his tent as they had an emergency generator there. The ice appeared and by then it was time to get up anyway for the safari.

On the safari I said to Bob that I thought he was very good when he came to see Mick in the early hours. Bob told me that he had never treated a scorpion sting in his life! 'Well, you have a very good bedside manner' I replied. We have since learned that there are over 1,700 species of scorpion in the world, all having a venomous sting but the vast majority do not represent a serious threat to humans. Healthy adults do not need any medical treatment after being stung and only 25 species have venom capable of killing a human. In some parts of the world with highly venomous species human fatalities

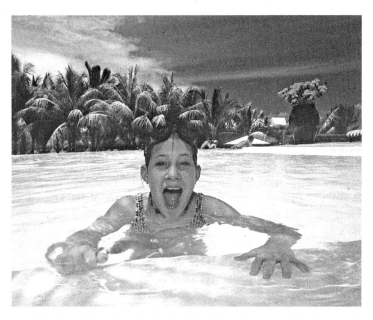

Figure 11.5 Granddaughter Rosie in Mauritius for the millennium: all our grandchildren are good swimmers.

occur regularly, especially in areas with limited access to medical treatment. Scorpions are ground-dwelling, tree-living rock and sand-loving. The oldest fossil scorpion dates from 430 million years ago. They are nocturnal, emerging at night to hunt and feed. And presumably to sting heroes like Mick.

12 More on work trips to Greece, Italy and Spain

Until the lock down began on 23 March, almost 11 weeks ago, I usually travelled abroad once or twice a month, mostly for work, including conferences, workshops, teaching and business meetings. I have visited 103 of the 192 independent countries in the world, and in this chapter I am singling out Europe, more precisely Greece, Spain and Italy where I have had some wonderful holidays as well as work experiences.

One memorable visit involved a summer school at which I taught at Xylokastro in the Peloponnese in 2003. It was organised by a man from the International Neuropsychological Society, Andy Papanicolau, an American, originally from Greece. Although the summer school was for a month, I said I would do the first two weeks and another guy could do the last two weeks (Jose Leon-Carrion was invited to do this). Mick came with me, we flew to Athens and then caught a bus to Xylokastro, to stay in a decent hotel with a reasonable swimming pool. Elizabeth Warrington was another presenter at the summer school (she gave a course on semantic memory) and the three of us joined up for most of our meals. Other courses the students could choose from were Memory and the Brain: Neuroanatomical and Functional Imaging: Correlates of Memory and Memory Disorders given by Hans Markowitsch; Neuropsychology of Amnesia Syndromes – Gianfranco Dalla Barba and Memory and Consciousness – Marcel Kinsbourne.

We loved the town which was on the coast with a forest along the shoreline. The townspeople were very welcoming and the mayor arranged some special events. We had the mornings free to swim and explore and I worked for two hours every afternoon, Monday to Friday, on different aspects of memory rehabilitation. It was a fantastic experience and some of the students who came to my sessions have been friends for life, including Dana Wong from Australia who is now a senior lecturer at La Trobe University in Melbourne and Anna Adlam who is currently an associate professor at the University of

Exeter. Anna had just completed her PhD at the time and would be coming to work at the unit in Cambridge where I was then employed. Anna's father, Richard, came to visit her and took her to Mycenae and Delphi at the weekends. Mick and I were invited to join them. We had two wonderful trips to these important historic places. Delphi is especially beautiful set along the slopes of Mount Parnassus, the site of the ancient oracle, filled with beautiful buildings, walls and monuments. It was established in the eighth century BC and was regarded as the centre of the world. Mick and I were impressed with the beauty, the intense blue light of the place and the tremendous views of mountain landscapes. Mycenae was quite different but immensely impressive and extraordinarily well ordered, a prehistoric site dating from 1600 to 1100 BC. It was the first advanced civilisation in mainland Greece and had its own writing system. It was dominated by an elite warrior class and became the setting of much ancient Greek literature. Anna is now on the committee of our Special Interest Group in Neuropsychological Rehabilitation and also reviews many of the papers on child neuropsychology submitted to our journal.

There have been other memorable trips to Greece, the last being in 2019 for three conferences organised by Elepap, a Greek organisation with the English translation of the acronym standing for Rehabilitation for Disabled People. The first conference was in Athens, the second in Thessaloniki and the third in Ioannina. The main focus of Elepap's work is with children and we visited some fantastic places providing rehabilitation for disabled children. The meetings as well as the hospitality were invariably good. I gave three presentations, with these being repeated at each city. The first was on 'general principles of neuropsychological rehabilitation'. The second on 'memory rehabilitation' and the third on 'the past, present and future of neuropsychological rehabilitation'. We also had time to visit the Parthenon in Athens, the market in Thessaloniki and Lake Pamvotid in Ioannina. We had visited Ionannina two or three years earlier. Prior to that visit, Mick and I had agreed that when we were there we would try to reach a small village in the mountains where Mick had worked for the International Voluntary Service way back in 1959. The village where he had worked 57 years ago was in the mountains close to Ioannina and was then named Neon Amaroussion. However, whenever Mick and I looked for this place on a map of Greece we could only find one near Athens, not the same village at all. In 1959 Mick was there with several other volunteers involved in digging trenches and building a pipe line so that the villagers could get fresh water pumped to their village instead of walking miles with donkeys to fetch water in casks. It was appreciated that pumping water directly to villages in the mountains would be an historical achievement and would help villagers to join the twentieth century. Once we knew we were going to Ioannina we increased our efforts to find Neon Amaroussion and discovered that some time after 1959 the village changed its name to its original name, Doliani. Although unheard of elsewhere, apparently it is not impossible for villages to change their names in Greece! Well of course when we looked at the map we were able to find Doliani easily and subsequently arranged for a taxi to take us there one Sunday morning. In 1959 the village was fairly poor and was still suffering from years of Nazi occupation in the 1940s – which turned out to be bloody and relentless as the mountain villagers fought the occupiers. When Mick was camping in the village in 1959 with other volunteers from round the world there were several chests in the church filled with skeletons and skulls of freedom fighters who had lost their lives to the occupiers.

When the taxi, the driver of which was also our tour guide, arrived at the village on the Sunday morning many of the villagers seemed to be enjoying drinks under some magnificent trees in the village square. We settled down to a drink and then the guide turned to some villagers sitting at a table near us and apparently told them that Mick had been one of the volunteers who had worked there in 1959. Well, Mick has not often been a celebrity but we were soon surrounded by most of the villagers including the older ones who remembered 1959. One, in particular, was an elderly man who had been a schoolboy then. Many photos were taken and as a final gesture one of the villagers walked over to a very large pipe, turned on a tap and clear water came gushing out. We took a photo of this as we waved good bye from the taxi! Mick was impressed with the

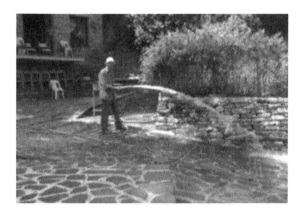

Figure 12.1 Water still being supplied to Doliani after 57 years.

laid back feel to the village with its well-dressed inhabitants in their Sunday best, contrasting with the poverty that existed in the village in 1959, all the women dressed in black then as standard dress for all occasions, working in the fields, and donkeys rather than the modern cars parked there now.

Italy and Spain are other Mediterranean countries I love and I have given lectures and workshops in both. One of my precious memories is a conference held in Padova, Italy, many years ago. The lecture theatre we were meant to be in had to close for some reason and we were directed to another theatre. Once we were all seated, the chairman said 'Ladies and gentlemen, I want you to know that Galileo Galilei once lectured in this room'. That sent a thrill through me as I began my talk. I was keeping good company!

I have visited many Italian cities, nearly every one a treasure because Italian architecture is superb. My favourite city in the world is prob-ably Siena in Tuscany which I went to in 1982 after a conference in Chianciano Terme. Siena has splendid fourteenth-century architecture around the Piazza del Campo where the famous horse race, The Palio, is held every year. The campanile throws a shadow around the Piazza like a sundial.

The conference in Chianciano Terme was the first meeting of the International Neuropsychological Society that I ever attended (I was to become president of this society from 2006 to 2007). I flew to Pisa, stayed the night there and the following morning I took the train to Chianciano Terme, famous for its thermal baths. At the railway station I asked for a ticket to the town which I pronounced as if it were an English word, the ticket master made me say the name correctly before selling me the ticket! He did this in a very sweet way though and made me smile. Once at the meeting I spoke about lateralisation of sign language in deaf people as this had been the research I undertook for my clinical psychology mas-ter's degree. I met many people there including a number from the United Kingdom and thought how strange that these worked so close to me at home yet I had to travel overseas to meet them. One American there, Manfred Maier (who died in 2006), came to me after my talk and asked why I had used British subjects? I am a British psychologist, working in the UK so obviously my participants were British and I thought what a strange question to ask. I realised later that he was confusing me with the American Barbara Wilson. In the first memoirs book I talk about the confusions there had been between the two of us and this question in Italy was yet another example of that.

I will mention another Italian meeting in Pavia in Northern Italy organised by Caterina Pistarini who is very active in the World

Federation of NeuroRehabilitation (WFNR). Our special interest group (SIG) in Neuropsychological Rehabilitation is affiliated to the WFNR. I am chair of this group and also chair of the chairs of the other 34 SIGS. We decided to have a meeting of all the chairs of the SIGS every two years and the first was held in Pavia in 2013. The second meeting was held in Abu Dhabi hosted by Sabahat Wasti, the third was in Shanghai in China hosted by Jianan Li and Tieban Yan. The most recent meeting in 2019 was held in Genoa, Italy and hosted once again by Caterina Pistarini. All the meetings were good but, being the first, the Pavia meeting was in some ways the most memorable and exciting. Each chair spoke for 10 minutes about his or her SIG and then there was a general and lively discussion. I felt our SIG was the most active as we hold a two-day international conference every year and we are the only SIG to do that. I also believe we publish more than other SIGS. In Pavia, we were taken from our hotel to the university and the meeting place each day by a little wooden train on wheels that was delightful. I remember a tour of the city where we saw a statue of Volta, credited with inventing the electric battery and from whom the words volt and voltage are derived. My last trip to Italy was in December 2019, just before the pandemic occurred. I was invited to speak in Bologna by Costanza Papagno, a neurologist with a PhD in neuropsychology. I had known Costanza since she worked in Cambridge with Alan Baddeley in the 1990s.

Spain is a country I feel I could live in as I love the food, the wine, the weather and the people. For a few years I have been going to Spain on average five times a year. We have a time share in Mallorca at the Marriott Resort in Son Antem, not too far from Palma and now own three weeks a year there. All the children, grandchildren and great grandchild have used it at some time or another but this chapter is about work and, of course, I frequently go to Spain for work too. In fact, as I write this, I am supposed to be at a meeting in Rioja but had to cancel because of the Covid-19 pandemic. My most recent award was the annual award from the Spanish Clinical Neuropsychology Society which I received in Barcelona in 2019. My closest colleague in Spain is Juan Carlos Arango Lasprilla, originally from Colombia, he now works in Bilbao, Northern Spain. He heard me present a workshop in Bogota, Colombia many years ago and said that was when he decided to specialise in brain injury rehabilitation. This is his memory of the workshop.

I don't recall the exact date, but you gave a course in Bogota on Neuropsychological Rehabilitation of Memory sometime between 1994–1996. At that time I was finishing my bachelor's degree in

Psychology at the University of Antioquia in Medellin. My brother had suffered a severe TBI due to a motorcycle accident. My dad has passed away and, as the oldest son, I became the primary financial caregiver for my family. I didn't have the funds to attend your course.

I called the course organizers to ask if they might be able to waive my registration fee if I helped to disseminate publicity concerning the course in my hometown of Medellin. They agree and I posted flyers in hospitals and rehabilitation centers throughout the city. With the registration fee waived, I had to figure out how to raise funds for the 10.5 hours bus trip from Medellin to Bogota.

One early form of crowd-sourcing funds that was common at that time (and still is) is to hold a raffle. I offered people the opportunity to buy tickets to win a small amount money, and any of the extra money from the ticket sales went towards my trip. In this way, I was able to raise enough funds to buy a round trip bus ticket.

I left Medellin at 6pm and got to Bogota at 5am. I went to the course. I didn't speak English at the time and took advantage of the simultaneous translation offered. During that course, hearing your passion for the topic, I realized that this was my calling. I wanted to become an expert in neuropsychological rehabilitation to help my brother and the many, many others throughout Latin America who were in similar circumstances. I hoped for the day that I might be able to collaborate more closely with you. Since I didn't have money for a hotel, once the course ended, I returned to Medellin via overnight bus trip that night.

One of the best meetings I ever attended was organised by Juan in Bilbao in 2016. This was the Iberoamerican Congress of Neuropsychology. There were 1,400 attendees and over 50 speakers from more than 25 countries around the world. Juan had persuaded some eminent speakers to come including Don Stuss from Toronto (who sadly died in September 2019). I wrote an obituary for Don which appeared in The Neuropsychologist (Wilson 2020c). Don was best known for his work on frontal lobes and I spoke about this in the obituary but I also told more personal things. Don's father was Ukrainian and Don never forgot this heritage. He spoke Ukrainian and was knowledgeable about his heritage. He was an enthusiast for many things, not just neuropsychology. Don, my husband, Mick, and I shared a keen interest in Shakespeare and the three of us visited the Shakespeare festival in Stratford, Ontario one year. Don met us at Toronto airport and drove us to Stratford. On the way he said we needed to stop for breakfast and he took us to a Macdonald's. I never go to Macdonald's as I boycott this chain for various reasons. However, I did not want to be impolite so went and chose the least Macdonaldy thing I could think of for breakfast (a fish burger). As we were leaving I admitted to Don that I had only gone to be well mannered. He was very amused and insisted we order some take out coffee in a Macdonald's bag which he then made me carry and photographed me doing this. I remember his infectious laugh to this day as he pointed out that he now had photographic evidence of my love of Macdonald's!

Back to the meeting in Bilbao: this was the first time that professionals interested in neuropsychology from Spain, Portugal and Latin America were going to be able to come together in a large Spanish-speaking event. At the time, Juan Carlos was working at the University of Deusto, who did not think he could bring so many people together. They offered him inadequate space that was unsuitable for such a big event. When the registrations started coming in and it was clear how much interest had been generated, Juan Carlos lost favour with the university with some colleagues boycotting the event and spreading negative publicity. Four or five months before the congress, Juan Carlos was forced to change the venue and organise it with the help of three of his students. The meeting was a huge success and in fact, since then, bi-annual congresses have been held with the fourth congress planned for 2021. Each Congress has had over 800 participants. So Juan Carlos most definitely proved the university wrong. Of course, all the speakers were taken to visit the famous Guggenheim Museum which Bilbao is most well known for.

Juan Carlos Arango Lasprilla and I have also given a course on rehabilitation together in India and a two day workshop in Alicante in 2019. Recently, together with Laiene Olabarrieta Lancia we published a book in Spanish (Arango Lasprilla, Wilson & Olabarrieta Lancia 2020). Although published in March 2020, it is unobtainable as it is still with the publishers in Mexico because of the coronavirus pandemic.

Before leaving this section on Spain, I feel I have to mention the eruption of the Icelandic volcano Eyjafjallajökull in April 2010 as I was in Mallorca giving a lecture at the university there when this happened. I gave my lecture and was planning to come home the next day to spend three days at home before Mick and I were setting off for a special cruise in Western Australia. We were going to see ancient aborigine art, swim with whale sharks and have a fantastic time. This was not to be, however. I returned to the hotel in Palma and telephoned Mick who told me I might not be able to return home as there had been a volcanic eruption in Iceland and planes were not allowed to fly in many places round the world. At first I thought I would be OK as I am a natural optimist but early next morning I went on line to find out just what was happening. There were no flights back to the UK but there were domestic flights within Spain. I was still hoping to get back home in time to do the Australian trip so I put my thinking cap on and decided to fly to the mainland as I would have a better chance of getting home from there.

I checked out of the hotel and took a bus to the airport. I asked the bus driver how much it cost to get to the airport and he said 'dos euros', I could not believe it was only two euros and thought he meant 'doce (twelve) euros' but, no, it really was only two euros. Once at the airport, I saw large numbers of people sitting on the floor waiting for news of flights (some did not get home for a week). I went to the Iberia office and managed to get a flight that morning to Barcelona. Once there I went straight to the railway station to try to book a train to Paris from where I hoped to get the Eurostar to the UK. Unfortunately, there were no trains available and I was advised to go to the bus station. I went there and joined a very long queue. Eventually, I reached the front of the queue and was told the next available bus to Paris was the following evening. I felt sick as it was so close to the time we should be departing for Australia but I booked the ticket on the night bus to Paris. I thanked my lucky stars that I wasn't poor and could do this and that I was an experienced traveller who could solve problems. The next thing was to find a hotel for the night and there was an information office nearby to help book. I did this and as I was walking past the ticket office I saw and heard an Australian woman struggling at the ticket desk. My Spanish isn't good but I have enough to scrape by (as a rule). I went to help and it appeared she had already paid for her ticket but the man was asking for more. I explained in my limited Spanish that she had paid and he explained that there was a surcharge. I told her this, she paid up and, after thanking me for my help, went on her way. I went to the hotel, emailed Mick to keep him in touch and went on line to try to book a ticket on Eurostar from Paris to London. Unfortunately, there were no seats left on any of the trains departing that would fit in with my bus arriving in Paris. So I had to think again. I found a ferry departing from Calais that had seats and I worked out I could get a train from Paris to Calais and then take the ferry to Dover, a train to London, another to Cambridge and another to Bury St Edmunds or I could get Mick to meet me in Dover. I paid for the ferry in order to ensure a place. I realised we would probably miss our flight to Australia though. Then I decided to go on line again and check Eurostar once more. Luckily, I found that extra trains had been put on and I could get a seat after all. So I paid for that seat and had to write off the ferry ticket which I no longer needed.

I took the overnight bus from Barcelona to Paris which wasn't as bad as I feared. I managed to get some sleep and there were stops for toilets. I took a cab from the bus station in Paris to Gare du Nord where the Eurostar leaves from. There was a wait there, so I walked around and had breakfast until it was time to queue for the train, board and find my seat. The train journey was straightforward and I knew my way home from St Pancras. So I arrived home just in time to pack for the journey to Australia but there were no flights going from Heathrow either so we never made the trip. Fortunately, most of the money was refunded through insurance and I did appear on BBC Look East on the lunchtime news explaining my journey. I was dropped from the main evening news though as another story was considered more interesting! I have remained proud of my involved exploits to get home from Spain and thus avoid horrible, dispiriting delays stuck in the initial airport for days, which was the fate of others less travel-wise than myself. I think it would be fair to say I am a seasoned traveller who knows her way round the world!

13 Other work trips to Cuba, New Zealand, Argentina and South Africa

I have been to Cuba only once, for a conference in 1998. We had to take a roundabout route because the USA at that time had an embargo which prevented flights between the States and Cuba. So we had to fly from Miami to Jamaica and then from Jamaica to Cuba, a most circuitous way of getting there! As usual, I took my jewellery in hand luggage and there was such a fuss at immigration in Havana, assuming, I think, that it had been stolen, that on the return journey I foolishly put the jewellery in my check-in luggage only to have it stolen from there! It included the beautiful necklace I had bought in Zanzibar two years earlier! I could not claim on insurance as this does not cover jewellery placed in check-in bags! We spent a few days in Havana, the capital of Cuba and a potentially stunning city but very run down because of the effects of the American embargo. For example, one of the men we met said he had trained as an airline pilot in Russia but now had to work as a taxi driver as there was no work for him in the aviation industry.

Despite the obvious poverty, there were good things about Cuba. Everywhere one stopped, whether it was a café, restaurant, park or whatever, musicians came to play and dancers danced. The sense of fun was palpable: the colours vibrant, the sounds made even me want to dance, and the well preserved ancient cars were a joy to see actually working.

The conference was in Varadero, a beautiful resort area. I don't remember much about the meeting itself but for one incident when I noticed all the men, including Mick, were queueing up round some tall bushes in the hotel garden. I found out they were buying Cuban cigars, that were illegal to take into the USA – even if you were flying back via Jamaica as we were to find out, when we had to stop overnight in Miami on our way home. We were aware that we were not supposed to take Cuban cigars into the USA but we were in transit and only there for one night so I assumed we would be OK. When we were going through Customs in Miami, the officer asked directly if we had bought any cigars. It is difficult for either of us to lie so we admitted to having a box of 20. We explained we were going home the next day but the officer sent us downstairs to the customs area for a more serious enquiry. The man there was more understanding and was not interested in fining us as we were definitely going to take the cigars home to Britain. He actually joked about the 'idiot' from upstairs who had sent us to him! (Somehow, I feel that such humanity is now missing from the USA in the year 2020.) As we left to go to the hotel Mick said to the officer, 'I bet your president has Cuban cigars'. The guy said, 'I don't know if he smokes them but I sure know where he puts them!' I needn't explain the reference to what was then the recent Bill Clinton and Monica Lewinsky affair!

New Zealand is a beautiful country which I do not know as well as Australia but I have been there a few times. At the present time they have a president, Jacinda Ardern, whom I really admire. I first went to New Zealand in 1993 when Jim Bolger was president. I flew from the USA where I had been at yet another conference, to give a talk in Auckland. I stayed with Dorothy Gronwall, best known for her work on the PASAT (Paced Auditory Serial Addition Test). Some people think she invented the test but she always made it clear she did not invent it although she did a fair amount of research on it. Sadly Dorothy, a delightful person, died in 2001 at the age of 70 years.

Mick did not come to New Zealand with me, although he was in the USA from where I flew to NZ. He flew home from Los Angeles. My mother was very ill and likely to die, she was in a nursing home near Southampton having been ill with vascular dementia for several years. I just hoped she would stay alive long enough for me to get home. I stayed with Dorothy and gave my talk at the university. I had to fly home via the USA and spend one night at an airport hotel there. I phoned Mick who told me my mother had just died. I was upset, it was too sudden, I wanted to grieve, thinking if only I had been a day earlier! Mick said he had seen her and she would not have recognised me but I felt that wasn't the point. I wanted to say goodbye. He met me at Heathrow and we drove straight to Southampton where we were guided through everything. My poor mum! This was so different from the situation when Sarah died in the year 2000. Losing a child is the worst thing that can happen; losing a mum is less tragic; at least it's the right way round.

I have had some happy experiences in New Zealand with our friends Kay and Tommy Farrar from Wellington and have another good friend Jenni Ogden, once a well-known neuropsychologist and now a writer of fiction. Jenni and her husband, John, have a house on the wonderful Great Barrier Island near Auckland. I stayed with them in 2008 when I happened to be training for the London Marathon. One day I spent running 20 miles along a beautifully sandy beach, quite hard surfaced. John drove to the end point and was waiting for me when I finished.

One of the INS meetings was held in Auckland in July 2013 and afterwards we had a SIG meeting in Rotorua where I saw a real-life kiwi. The bird is bigger than I was expecting. In New Zealand at the beginning of a meeting the Maoris sing a welcoming song. This is often an emotional experience. At the INS meeting in New Zealand Erin Bigler was to give the opening address and cried when he was sung to. I had a similar experience in New Zealand a year or two later when I was giving a workshop in Auckland: the Maori women sang me in with a special song for '*the respected older woman*' I felt a little bit uncertain about that but, no, it was a lovely thing for them to do.

Another country I find very beautiful is Argentina. I first went there to give a lecture in the capital, Buenos Aires, in 1984 not that long after the war in the Falklands or the Malvinas as the Argentinians call the islands. Mick and I hated that war which took place in 1982, we have heard it described as 'two bald men fighting over a comb'. Mick was playing in a jazz band in 1982 and afterwards the band never played together again. I'll explain. At that time our country was split between those who supported Maggie Thatcher's decision to go to war and those who were opposed to such action. The pub landlord, where the band played each week, wanted the band to do a special session in support of the British soldiers. Half the band were in favour of the idea and half were not. So the event never took place, the landlord refused to continue with the regular Thursday nights, and the band never played together again. War can be ruinous!

We were nervous about going to Argentina as we thought there would be an anti-British feeling but we did not experience this at all. We were well treated, my lecture was appreciated and, at the times when we did discuss the war, the Argentinians reassured us there was no animosity towards the United Kingdom. They seemed to appreciate the fact that we ensured the end of the military Junta which was over-thrown in December 1983. We loved Buenos Aires which reminded us of Paris with its architecture although we were saddened by the women who marched around the Plaza de Mayo every Thursday in memory of the disappeared. Wikipedia (downloaded 7 June 2020) says

> Women had organized to gather, holding a vigil, while also trying to learn what had happened to their adult children during the

1970s and 1980s. They began to gather for this every Thursday, from 1977 at the Plaza de Mayo in Buenos Aires, in front of the Casa Rosada presidential palace, in public defiance of the government's law against mass assembly. Wearing white head scarves to symbolise the diapers (nappies) of their lost children, embroidered with the names and dates of birth of their offspring, now young adults, the mothers marched in two's in solidarity to protest the denials of their children's existence or their mistreatment by the military regime. Despite personal risks, they wanted to hold the government accountable for the human rights violations which were committed in the Dirty War.

After the lecture in Buenos Aires Mick and I had a few days in Salta and Molinos. We hired a driver and loved the beautiful mountains. We have also visited Mendoza where Malbec wine is made and I have visited Ushuaia, the capital of Tierra del Fuego way down in the south of the country. This is where I boarded the ship to go to Antarctica.

In many ways my strongest link in Argentina is with Córdoba in central Argentina near the foothills of the Sierras Chicas on the Suquía River. I was given an honorary degree from the university of Córdoba in 2014. The person who initiated this was Andrea Querejeta, a psychologist I have come to admire. The old part of the university is beautiful and I loved the degree ceremony which was very traditional. I also gave a lecture there.

Andrea Querejeta came to my rescue in 2018. I received an email from a young woman I had never heard of asking me to present a two-day workshop in Córdoba. We discussed the airfare and the honorarium and agreed that I would buy the ticket and this would be refunded when I had given the workshop. I checked three times that if I bought the ticket it would be refunded and three times was reassured so I purchased it. Then about two weeks before I was due to go to Argentina, the woman emailed me to say the workshop had been cancelled! I was shocked and said I needed the money for the ticket to be refunded. The woman emailed back saying 'No tengo dinero' (I don't have money). I tried British Airways who would not refund the money. In a panic I emailed Andrea Querejeta and asked if she could do anything. I knew I would lose money but anything she could do would be appreciated. Bless her, Andrea arranged a one-day workshop for me at short notice and agreed to refund some of the money. I went to Córdoba, had a very good time and the workshop seemed to go well. I asked Andrea what she thought when she received my email explaining how my money was lost. She said she nearly had a heart attack. So this is another country I like but the economy is not good and they are still suffering from the effects of the Junta, as I witnessed when I came across a whole street in Córdoba filled with photographs of the disappeared.

The final country I want to mention in this chapter is South Africa, which I have already described as one of our favourites for safaris. However, I have also given lectures, workshops and conferences there. My last trip to South Africa with Sarah was to Durban in 1999 at a mid-year meeting of the INS. After the conference we went to Cape Town and from there to Robben Island, where Nelson Mandela had been imprisoned for many years. A very special and thought provoking place.

A friend and colleague from Cape Town, one of the world's most beautiful cities, is Leigh Schrieff. I remember meeting her at a conference in Cape Town in 2008 and then at NR-SIG meetings after that. At the meeting in Rotorua, New Zealand she was so helpful and kind to Pauline Monro who had difficulties walking because of her mobility problems. It was Leigh to whom I owe gratitude for a debate in which I participated in South Africa at an international psychology meeting in 2012. I had agreed to give one of the keynote addresses for which I had prepared and then, about three weeks before the congress was due to start I had an email from Leigh saying she was looking forward to my debate with Mark Solms. I panicked having completely forgotten I had agreed to do this. I checked up and indeed I had agreed.

The debate was entitled 'Are psychoanalysis and neuropsychology incompatible?' I worked hard for the next three weeks preparing for this debate. I knew Mark Solms had worked in London with Michael Kopelman so I emailed Mike to see if he could give me any advice. He emailed back 'Oh, my god'. This did not fill me with hope. Several people told me it would be difficult debating with Mark Solms especially on his own territory. In the end I need not have worried as I thought I did a good job which was well rewarded by the response of the audience.

The hall was packed. Mark went first and had no slides. He was unprepared, without notes, very relaxed, hands in pockets and extremely confident. His main theme was that the psychology was missing from neuropsychology as neuropsychologists did not deal with emotional problems! That is, of course, far from the truth as I made clear in my disputation. I was, as always, well prepared with copious slides and detailed notes. Also, I had taken time to read and check on Solms' work. I am not a supporter of psychoanalysis as there seems to be no way of confirming or disconfirming any statements made. For example, a patient reported in a paper by Solms (1995) had sustained a right hemisphere stroke with unilateral neglect (failure to report, respond or orient to stimuli on one side of space) and left hemiplegia. Such patients are sometimes unaware of, or indifferent to, their difficulties. This particular patient suffering from depression, hated her left arm However, said Solms, because her attachment to her own body had necessarily been a narcissistic one, her attitude towards these introjected lost objects was decidedly ambivalent. This part of her own beloved self, which she had naturally assumed was under her omnipotent control, had suddenly revealed itself to be a piece of external reality after all – and moreover, it had revealed itself to be an unreliable piece of reality, an object which she needed and loved, but which had nevertheless abandoned her. Her constant refrain that 'everybody hates me' therefore turned out to be a projection of an internal situation in which a previously healthy and independent part of herself was hated by a now-crippled and dependent part of herself. Her hatred of this introjected image of her lost self could be traced back analytically to its infantile origins in her identification with her mother, that is, it could be traced back to her identification with the woman upon whom she had depended for so long during childhood (Solms 1995).

This made me angry and I argued 'How does he KNOW this? How does he know if he is right or wrong? What other explanations might there be?' For example, her 'hated' arm may have represented her disability or, it might have been because of problems with body image or due to the location of the brain lesion. As scientists we have to prove or disprove any theories we have to explain patients' behaviour. I argued strongly for the scientific approach, and gave plenty of examples. I felt I had won the debate although there was not a vote. I certainly had some positive feedback afterwards.

I have made several trips to South Africa and had some very successful meetings there. My last trip was in July 2019 when I gave a lecture at Witwatersrand University at the invitation of Sahba Besharati. I have also given a lecture there the year before and had been given a private tour of the Cradle of Mankind Museum, which is remarkably beautiful and informative in terms of its presentation of scientific and social information about the natural environment, the people, places and artefacts of South Africa.

In 2019, Sahba arranged for me to give a talk at the Nelson Mandela Hospital in Johannesburg. What an honour that was! Rachel Everett, one of our administrators wrote a short piece for the OZC newsletter. Barbara Wilson gave a talk at The Nelson Mandela Children's Hospital in Johannesburg on the Assessment and Management of People with a Disorder of Consciousness. This was organised by Dr Sahba Besharati, a neuropsychologist. After a tour of the wonderfully well-equipped hospital, Barbara gave a one and a half hour lecture which was well attended by a mixed audience of a large variety of professionals and well received.

14 Learning from patients

I firmly believe that I have learned a great deal from patients. Not only did I realise very early on that treatment techniques I learned in my training had to be modified for survivors of a brain injury, I also learned that some things I held as truths had to be changed as a result of the views of patients with whom I worked. One of the best examples is Kate, whom I have known for many years and from whom I learned many things. I often think of Kate as a true heroine and I am proud to say we have published together (Wilson, Gracey & Bainbridge 2001; Wilson & Bainbridge 2014). Kate's recovery has lasted many years and, would appear to be continuing, albeit very slowly, even though she developed ADEM (Acute Disseminated Encephalomyelitis) in 1997 (Wilson 2019). Kate is an important person in many ways and she changed my thinking in one very significant respect.

In the UK one can apply to the courts for permission to remove food and water from a patient if there is no evidence of cognition and I thought that this was perfectly acceptable until Kate, who had survived a very severe brain injury, was adamant that we should not let her and others like her die in this manner. I came to realise that mistakes can be made, as Wilson and Betteridge (2019) describe. Since getting to know Kate in 1999, I have marked reservations about removing food and water from such patients and believe a civilised society should care for those who cannot make decisions for themselves. Living wills are not the answer either as people change their minds after becoming ill (ibid.). Back to Kate and what happened to her.

Kate was a teacher when she became ill in 1997 with acute ADEM, an autoimmune kind of encephalitis. She had damage to her brainstem and both thalami. She had a disorder of consciousness for several months. She was one of the very first patients in a vegetative state to have a PET scan (Menon et al. 1998). Her responses to photographs of familiar faces differed from responses to scrambled images with the same colours and brightness and the results were no different from those of an age-matched control. When Kate left hospital 22 months after becoming ill, her family was told that any further recovery was unlikely. At that time, Kate could make hardly any noise and had very little movement. She received eight years of neuropsychological rehabilitation where she was seen, on average, once every two weeks for about two hours at a time. Since then she has been seen once or twice each year to monitor her recovery. We are also in email contact regularly. The first paper about her (Wilson et al. 2001) demonstrated that Kate had normal cognitive functioning, and the second (Macniven et al. 2003) described treatment for her emotional difficulties. Wilson and Bainbridge (2014) describe her story in detail. She was last seen in early 2020. She remains physically impaired, she is in a wheelchair, is tube-fed and has a tracheostomy in place. However, she is cognitively normal and has used a computer for many years. She received speech therapy for six years. This was stopped as it was thought she would show no more change. Kate used to rely on a letter board to communicate but, determined to talk, threw this away after 14 years. She now communicates with perfectly intelligible speech. Recovery has slowed but has not completely stopped.

If Kate is in a low mood she might email me and I try to cheer her up by telling her what a special person she is and how she is my heroine. I do not believe I would be as strong as her if I had gone through the same trials she has survived. Her sense of humour is enviable and she frequently makes me smile. I once asked her why she had done so well and she said it was her Viking genes which made her so determined. She also has a passion for earrings and buys many pairs to cheer her up, especially during this lockdown. Here are some recent emails between Kate and me.

April 20th 2020 (from Kate to me)
Dear Barbara
Just thinking about where the Viking DNA comes from and my mum has it from her dad, my grandpa, and he was so determined.
I will never forget his determination, he was also just like Emma's father in Jane Austen's book Emma. He said things like him, he was a GP and a bit old fashioned and Emma's father makes me laugh as he is so like my grandpa. I love that book, it might be my favourite book as it reminds me of him so much. He was a Viking, his grandpa came from the Welsh board and his mum was Irish (she sounds a very strong woman). Just my thoughts on the Viking bit of me and you make me think of where it came from.
Love Kate

May 11th 2020 (from Kate to me

Dear Barbara

Hope all is OK for you in this lockdown.

I have been ordering earrings at least once a week, just ordered a pair after hearing no big change in the lockdown.

I always, after I get new pair, say this will be my last even almost believe it myself, but it only lasts a few days. So the last few weeks I have given up saying that as I know I will get more.

My mum read in the paper that in lockdown the sale of Amazon had gone up a lot and it is not just me!

Love Kate

May 11th 2020 (from me to Kate)

You are still funny Kate. I am definitely going to tell the story about you and your earrings in my next book.

Stay well

From your friend and admirer

Barbara

May 11th 2020 (from Kate to me)

Dear Barbara

I have another obsession John Lewis plain flannels. They are thick and soft, really nice on your, skin. I ordered some and they came today so am looking forward to washing my face tonight! Used to have loads, but in the lockdown I went through my flannels and binned them all and I really noticed. No other make is so soft and thick, only John Lewis flannels for me. My carer at the moment laughs at my earring obsession, she pointed out that I had 62 pairs!

Love Kate

May 29th 2020 (from Kate to me)

Dear Barbara

Hope all is OK for you with this lockdown, it feels normal to me now. When I have to go out it will seem odd and hard work. Like Dolly it is nice not having to go out, but rather boring. I really need a hair cut and to go shopping. Just ordered some more earrings, they were cheap (the postage cost more than the earrings) and just right so I had to buy them! Now for the last 3 weeks, I only got 1 pair a week, I want to say I won't buy any more but I said that the last 3 weeks when I got a pair. After I said I won't buy anymore, my carer said not this week! Its Friday so I thought I will not get any more this week, but I can never be 100% sure! It's the answer to this lockdown and my mum read in the paper that sales of Amazon earrings has gone up lots and it's not just me.

Love Kate

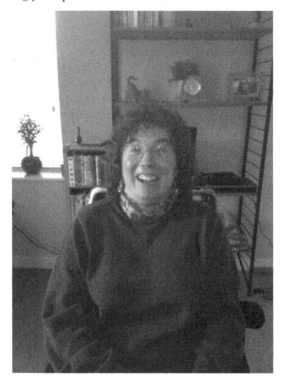

Figure 14.1 Kate at home.

Before we leave Kate, I want to tell one more story which might also illustrate a male-dominated approach. The Cambridge Coma Study group published a study some years ago showing that some people in a vegetative state could show a response when in a brain scanner (Owen et al. 2006). They were asked to imagine walking round a room or imagine playing tennis. Being vegetative, they could not speak or respond to the environment but in the scanner, the parts of the brain lighting up when asked to do these imaginary tasks were not statistically different from controls. This was such a revolutionary finding that the BBC decided to make a news item out of it. They wanted to find someone who had been in a vegetative state and recovered. I put them in touch with Kate and I was filmed translating for her as she was still using her letter board at that time. When it was shown on BBC, Adrian Owen, senior author was named with his name shown on the screen, so was the head of neurosurgery and the others carrying out the study. All were named but I was not! I had gone to some trouble to set this up. Kate had kindly agreed to take part but I was not named at all. I was not pleased and will never know if it was because I was a woman or because they felt I was unimportant in the story or for some other reason.

In addition to Kate, almost every patient is special and has something to teach us: one of the patients I saw with Anita Rose and her assistant Bethan Roberts, while working at the Raphael, was a man with environmental dependency syndrome (EDS). We presented this at a meeting in Cape Town (Roberts et al. 2018). This syndrome manifests itself with an array of symptoms including imitation behaviour, utilisation behaviour, and inappropriate responses to cues in the environment leading to the term 'Environmental Dependency Syndrome'. Lhermitte (1983; 1986) named the syndrome, describing it as an elaborate manifestation of utilisation behaviour but guided by the cues provided by the environment. Others such as, Archibald, Kerns, Mateer and Ismay (2005) and Ghosh and Dutt (2010) report the syndrome in children and in people with frontotemporal dementia. It has also been described in neuropsychiatric disorders (Marin & Gorovoy 2014). Patients with EDS are described as reaching out and automatically using objects in the environment in an 'object-appropriate' manner that is inappropriate for the particular context. For example, in a neuropsychological testing session, a patient with EDS might automatically pick up the tester's pen and paper on a table and begin writing something without being told or asked to do so. EDS has been associated with lesions of different brain areas (Lhermitte, Pillon, & Serdaru 1986); Ishihara, Nishino, Maki, Kawamura, & Murayama, S. 2002; Lagarde et al. 2013).

EDS in the context of rehabilitation can affect attention to task thus impeding on interventions both physical and cognitive reducing positive outcome of any treatment. Jessica Fish also came to see the patient and contribute to our discussions about the best way to treat our particular patient. We will call him Kevin (not his real name). We used a single case experimental design to investigate whether the frequency of Kevin's grasping of objects in his environment, could be reduced.

Kevin was 57 years old. In 2016 he sustained a brain haemorrhage following a period where he suffered several headaches. He was admitted to his local hospital with what was considered to be a mild stroke and then discharged. He deteriorated and returned to the same hospital later. A CT scan indicated a bleed and an aneurysm which was clipped. A repeat scan a few days later showed a large area of damage in the right hemisphere together with hydrocephalus. This required a ventriculoperitoneal (VP) shunt insertion. He had one seizure soon after surgery but no further seizures after that. He was left with physical difficulties, so was assessed in a wheelchair, together with cognitive deficits and some behavioural problems. He was referred for a neuropsychological assessment and seen on six occasions for an average of 30 minutes each session. He spoke quietly and kept his head turned to the right. He began the first session by asking for a kiss. When asked what he thought his main problems were he said 'problems with opposite sex'. On the whole, though, he cooperated with the assessment. The conclusions to the initial assessment were as follows

1   This is a man of least average premorbid ability. The Test of Premorbid Functioning may well underestimate his basic ability as he failed some items because of neglect. He also gave up on the last items.
2   He has a severe neglect of the left hand side of space (associated with right hemisphere damage). Not only is this evident on tests, but Mr XX keeps his head turned to the right.
3   He also has a significant retrograde amnesia.
4   His memory is poor.
5   Finally, he shows evidence of the environmental dependency syndrome (also known as utilisation behaviour). This means he is likely to grab anything in the environment and use it even when it is not his or not part of the task in hand. For example, whenever he is wheeled into the neuropsychology office, he grabs the umbrella or the walking stick in the right hand corner and tries to use it; if a pen is on the table he will pick it up and try to write something.

It was thought that giving Kevin something to hold would stop his constant grabbing of anything in the environment so the pilot study, carried out in one session of 40 minutes, investigated whether or not this was the case. He was asked to describe a picture and for each five-minute chunk of time, measures were taken of his attempts to grab objects on the table in front of him while holding or not holding a pen. The results were as follows:

No pen = 4 grabs
Pen = 0 grabs
Pen = 0 grabs
No pen = 2 grabs
Pen = 0 grabs
No pen = 3 grabs

Consequently, it was considered that giving him something to hold would reduce his EDS. The treatment employed an ABABA (a reversal) single case experimental design.

The first baseline (A) consisted of observations of K.I's environmental dependency in a clinic rehabilitation session over 8 occasions.
The first treatment phase (B) involved providing Kevin with a 12 sided 'fiddle toy' during clinic sessions. This treatment phase was conducted over 11 sessions.
During the second baseline (A) the fiddle toy was removed.
The second treatment (B) phase was the same as the first.
Following the second treatment phase a final baseline (A) was taken.

We showed clearly that the fiddle toy was effective in reducing the frequency of his grabbling behaviour as can be seen in Figure 13.1.

EDS is very disruptive to a patient's involvement in rehabilitation. The constant grabbing and using things in the environment that do not belong to the patient prevents adequate assessment. A simple treatment strategy such as providing the person with EDS something to hold, can reduce the problem behaviours and increase attention to tasks. This is a simple, cheap and effective way of reducing such behaviours.

The third patient is Tracey and this description is from Wilson and Okines 2014 (with permission).

At the age of 27 years Tracey was in the gym showing her daughter how to do cartwheels when she fell and hurt her neck, back and ankle. For the next three days Tracey suffered from headaches and dizzy spells. She saw her general practitioner who prescribed pain killers for her headache. On the third night she had a seizure lasting more than an hour. She then fitted for three hours.

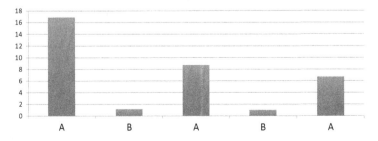

Figure 14.2 An ABABA design for treating a man with EDS.

Eventually, her boy friend called an ambulance and she was taken to hospital. A CT scan the following day showed something was wrong deep in Tracey's brain. She was transferred to another hospital for an MRI scan which showed that she had suffered a basilar artery thrombosis. A neurologist confirmed that the fall in the gym had probably caused a tear in the inner wall of the artery, which in turn caused clotting in the brain. Tracey went back to the original hospital where her parents were told she would probably not survive for more than a few months. Tracey's MRI scan found a large lesion in the pons (a structure in the brain stem). Some 90% of the pons was affected with slight sparing of extreme posterior section. The mid brain and thalami were not affected. There was no evidence of lesions in the cerebral hemispheres, particularly in temporal or parietal areas.

After a month in coma, Tracey began to regain consciousness. About four weeks later a nurse noticed that Tracey's eyes were following her as she moved around the room. Tracey's parents were told that their daughter was aware but her cognitive state was not known. A diagnosis of Locked-In Syndrome (LIS) was made. LIS is a rare consequence of brain damage. The condition is typically caused by a lesion in the pontine area (in the brain stem), usually a stroke in the basilar artery or a pontine haemorrhage. According to Schnakers et al 2008, at least 60 per cent of all cases fit this picture. Patients with LIS are fully conscious but unable to move or speak due to paralysis of nearly all voluntary muscles except the eyes.

Communication is with movement of the eyes. As Tracey became more alert she was able to answer questions by raising her eyes for 'Yes' and lowering them for 'No' allowing her parents to communicate with her. Her father accessed the internet and found information from the French Locked-in Syndrome Association (www.alis-asso.fr). A letter board was described using colours and letters. With some modifications, a similar board was made for Tracey and this is how people now communicate with her. The chart is organised with different colours on each row. Each row has certain letters and numbers. Thus, the first row is red and this has the letters A, B, C, D and 'end of word'; the second row is yellow and has the letters E, F, G, H and 'new word'; the third row is blue with the next set of letters and so forth. The last two rows are white depicting the digits 0–9.

First Tracey is asked to select the colour Red/Yellow/ Blue/ Green etc. When Tracey raises her eyes to the right colour we then say the letters (or digits) along that row until Tracey raises her eyes. Words are spelled out in this way. Tracey is very good at this. She does not need to actually see the board nor do those who communicate regularly with her as they can remember the colours and letters, but it is needed by others less familiar with the system.

Tracey has a tracheostomy tube in place, she is fed by a peg tube, she has hardly any movement apart from a little facial movement of her tongue and lips. This allows Tracey to make a small smile and she has limited head control. She is, however, alert and engaged. I first met her in January 2010. Her father, John and Angela, the speech and language therapist, showed me how to communicate with Tracey using the letter board. I had been asked to assess Tracey to see whether or not she had any problems with her memory, concentration, thinking and so forth. I knew about Locked-in Syndrome (LIS) and had assessed people who communicated with a letter board, but I had not assessed someone with LIS before. Because of this, I was very interested to meet Tracey and communicate with her. She was always cooperative and appeared to work to the best of her ability. I saw her two or three times a month until June 2010. Assessment was slow because of the communication method she was forced to use (Eyes raised for 'Yes' and lowered for 'No') and certain tests, such as tests of speed, motor functioning and recall of long passages could not be given. Nevertheless, many tests could be administered to her. It soon became apparent that Tracey had good concentration and an excellent working memory. She rarely forgot what word or sentence she was spelling and could keep in mind instructions given to her.

As well as tests of reasoning, memory perception and other cognitive tests, Tracey was assessed on a test of anxiety and depression, a scale to measure her perception of pain, and a test measuring her quality of life. Tracey did well on most tests. On two tests of executive functioning (problem solving and reasoning) she scored in the superior range of ability. This was also true of a test of verbal memory. She was good on tests of naming and language as well as basic visual perception and visual spatial processing. There were two areas where she appeared to have some difficulty: the first was in some aspects of visual memory and the second was with some more complex visual perception, visual organisation and visual reasoning tasks. This was thought to be due to the fact that she has some diplopia and blurring of vision making it difficult for her to scan complex arrays. She says her vision is 'like looking through the window of a moving vehicle with bad suspension'.

There was no suggestion that she was depressed or particularly anxious and Tracey, herself, agreed with this when the scores were fed back to her. On a pain rating scale, Tracey said she could feel pain normally anywhere in her body; she rated her headaches as 85 on a 0–100 scale and said she had this pain about 4 times a week. The pain was described as 'heavy and severe'. She believed her headaches were caused by her posture and a visiting pain expert said she thought this explanation was probably correct. Tracey's head is supported in a head rest, but due to her decreased head control and her strong cough reflex, when she coughs her head will fall forward causing increasing strain on the neck muscles. Since the pain assessment, Tracey has had rest breaks during the day and this has reduced the severity and frequency of her headaches.

On the quality of life measure, Tracey felt her general health was much better now than a year ago and she was experiencing far fewer respiratory infections. She did not rate herself as having any emotional problems and believes she has a reasonable quality of life. With Tracey's help we wrote a paper about LIS which was published in 2011 (Wilson et al 2011).

My conclusions to Tracey's assessment were as follows: emotionally, Tracey would appear to be a well balanced young woman with no serious cognitive difficulties and no obvious depression, anxiety or other mood issues despite the severe limitations placed on her because of her almost total paralysis.

Another striking finding from Tracey's history and other reports is the slow onset of the stroke leading to the LIS. It was several days since Tracey's original accident in the gym until the full blown paralysis and this is true of several other patients reported in the literature. The patient described by Garrard et al (2002) who had been to the hairdresser's, suffered neck pain, nausea, dizziness, clumsiness of the right arm and dysarthria and then five days later, a full blown stroke developed. These symptoms were very much like those described by Tracey. Other cases in the Garrard et al. (2002) paper also showed slow onset. Perhaps the case most similar to Tracey was a 37 year old woman who developed neck pain after slipping while standing on her head during yoga. Three days later she became paralysed and anarthric. Most strokes would appear to be of a much more sudden onset.

I saw Tracey again ten years after her stroke and four years after finishing rehabilitation, when she was seen in a residential home where she now lives. Her mobility, facial expressions and vocalisations were observed. With regard to mobility there were noticeable changes. She can now manoeuvre her electric wheelchair with head movements and has an environmental control system for switching on the television, opening the door and so forth. From an expressionless and motionless face caused by the accident, Tracey now has a very mobile visage with plenty of expressions: she can smile, laugh and express surprise. Despite the fact that most of her communications are with her eyes, she has some vocalisations. She can say 'hello' and 'thank you' but with difficulty.

We know from other studies that recovery does occur for some patients with LIS (Wilson, Allen, Rose, & Kubikova 2018). For the majority, however, LIS is complete and permanent despite some minor improvements. Tracey would fit into this category; she has made improvements but remains with a LIS. The chief evidence for this is that her main communication is with her eyes. What is not clear is how much more recovery could be achieved with more intensive rehabilitation.

These are just three of the many, fascinating patients I have seen over the years and I hope their stories help to convey reasons I am so committed to brain injury rehabilitation.

Just after writing this, I learned that Tracey, herself, has now written a book about her story and, soon, I hope to read it.

15   Brexit and Irish citizenship

Both Mick and I were so angry about leaving the European Community that we both decided to see if we could try to obtain Irish passports in order to remain Europeans. We knew that this was possible if we had a grandparent born in Ireland and, fortunately, we both had an Irish born grandmother and both our fathers were born of Irish mothers. Mick's grandmother had been born in Naas and mine in Dublin. We realised that if we were successful we would both own British and Irish passports and this seemed to us to be advantageous. Apart from the fact that Mick pointed out that he would never not be able to support the English rugby side we thought it would be a good idea to go ahead. We went for Mick's first as his seemed the most straightforward. In fact we decided to go for it during the referendum, just in case the unthinkable happened and Britain voted to leave. It took us ages to work out how to do it. One has to apply on line and first register as a foreign birth. Citizenship through a foreign birth has to be granted before one can apply for a passport. In order to go for this, one has to have the birth, marriage and death certificates of the grandparent born in Ireland and the parent who was born in the United Kingdom plus the birth and marriage certificates of the person applying. We searched our chest where we keep important papers and found some but not all of them. This meant we had to apply to Ireland for some of the certificates required and then to apply in England for others. Eventually we collected them all together, filled in the appropriate form on line, paid the registration fee (over 200 euros), and sent the certificates by registered post to Ireland. We waited for several months. It was a stressful procedure and we spent many hours on the computer working everything out.

Why didn't I apply at the same time you might ask? Well, as I said in Chapter 1, my father changed his name as a young man. This was the incident with the motor cyclist. I managed to find my dad's original

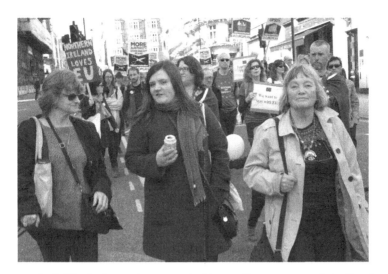

Figure 15.1 Jill, Jessica and me on the big pro-European march in London supported by over a million marchers.

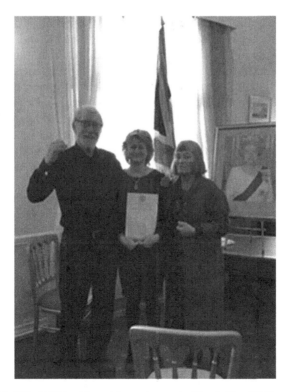

Figure 15.2 Jill's British citizenship ceremony in Cambridge 2018.

story in an old copy of the South London Press from, I think, the year 1928. There were many spelling mistakes in the original piece which I have rectified.

It said this:

> GIRL PILLION RIDER KILLED. A girl pillion rider was killed at Walthamstow yesterday. At p.m. Herbert John Palethorpe. aged 21, of Queen Elizabeth Walthamstow, was driving a motorcycle with Miss Florence Beatrice Smith (21), of Warner Road. Walthamstow, as a pillion passenger along Forest Road. Mr. Palethorpe collided with William Marsh, aged 16, of Norvillo Road, Walthamstow, who was alighting from a tram car in motion. The motorcycle struck Marsh, swerved into the kerb, and Miss Smith was thrown violently against a wall, receiving injuries from which she died almost immediately. Mr. Palethorpe was taken to Connaught Hospital with a fractured left shoulder, but was allowed go home. Marsh received slight injuries, and was medically attended on the spot.

Although my father received only a caution, he seemingly felt petrified to the extent that he felt he had to change his name and sort of disappear as William Marsh. Why he felt so bad when he was cleared of any crime is hard to understand. Mick and I have pondered over this many times and our only theory is that it might have been possible that my father thought that the injured parties were so incensed by the court's decision that they might try to 'get' him in revenge? We shall never know the reason, only my dad's reaction, which was to become William Forester for the rest of his life, including his fight against Hitler in the Second World War – which seemed to legitimise his change of name forever.

Coming back to my application for Irish citizenship, the Irish website stated that if a person involved had changed their name, evidence had to be provided for this such as a deed poll certificate or an old passport. As my father had done this illegally I thought this meant I would not be allowed to continue registering as an Irish citizen through a foreign birth and I procrastinated. Talking to an Irish friend, however, it was observed that so many people of Irish descent had changed their names that I should not worry. It was jokingly suggested that if I were challenged I should tell the person questioning me that my father had been fighting for the IRA! However, other Irish people said that under no circumstances should I say such a thing! Fortunately, my father's change of name was never questioned.

Meanwhile, after six months Mick received his registration of Irish citizenship via a foreign birth and was delighted. I still did nothing until the awful result of the Brexit referendum came through with the news that a tiny majority had won the vote to leave the European Union. I immediately went ahead to try for my foreign birth registration. By then I had collected together all the required certificates. I was a little worried about my Irish grandmother, as her birth certificate said Cathleen Welsh and her marriage and death certificates said Kathleen Walsh. The dates of birth and the parents' names, however, were the same. I sent my application off and had to wait 11 months because, by then so many people were applying for Irish citizenship. I had one email communication from the Irish office asking, not about my father's change of name as I had expected, but about my grandmother's name spelling. They simply wanted confirmation that it was the same person. I spoke again to my friend, who advised me to point out to the Dublin office that my grandmother's parents were illiterate and could not spell. As this was probably true, I replied reassuring the office that Cathleen Welsh and Kathleen Walsh were indeed the

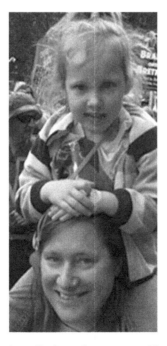

Figure 15.3 Granddaughter Rosie and great granddaughter Amélie on the London march.

same person. Eventually, my Irish citizenship came and, like Mick, I was delighted.

The next thing was to obtain our Irish passports which did not take as long as the foreign birth registration. Even here though, Mick's came a few weeks before mine. Because I had married and changed my name, I had a letter from the Irish passport office asking for my wedding certificate to prove I was the same person as in my birth certificate! Of course, I had sent all this for the original Irish citizenship and this had been returned but the passport office needed to see it too. I sent that off and, at last, my Irish passport came.

We had booked Easter in Spain and planned to use our new Irish passports in order to enter Spain as Europeans, but then the lockdown came and we were not able to fly! Three months later and we still haven't used our Irish passports. Will it ever happen? I say more about lockdown in Chapter 17. As for Brexit, we have recently learned that there is to be no extension and the transition period will definitely end in December despite many, many people thinking this is idiocy.

16 Coping with bereavement twenty years on

It is over 20 years now since Sarah died in a white water rafting accident in Peru, and, as members of The Compassionate Friends (TCF), the support group for bereaved families, say: 'we have learned to live with it'. We hardly ever cry now about Sarah although we still think about her every day, we talk about her, we refuse to make her death a taboo subject. We remember the African proverb we put in our 2004 book on coping with bereavement (Wilson & Wilson 2004) 'As long as you speak my name I shall live forever'. We celebrate Sarah's birthday and the anniversary of her death. We are never quite sure whether we should do this on the day she actually died, 12 May or the day we learned about her death, 15 May. Jon Evans as always, sends us a message remembering the event; the only member outside the family to do so. We were going to have a special memorial dinner for the 20-year anniversary of her dying and had booked a restaurant in Bury St Edmunds but the coronavirus pandemic came, we had lock down and all restaurants were closed. So members of the immediate family remembered Sarah in our weekly Zoom meeting and Carol, Sarah's aunt, left a bottle of bubbly for us on the doorstep. I describe life during lockdown in the next chapter, but will just say here that, like all citizens, we were not allowed to meet people who did not live with us for weeks: people who wanted to see us or had something to deliver, knocked on the door, and if they had something to leave, left whatever it was on the doorstep, before stepping back a few feet. We could then talk from a distance of two metres.

Zoom, a kind of upmarket Skype, became very important to many people as a result of the pandemic, including me, but more of this in the following chapter. Early on in the lockdown we arranged to have a weekly family meeting via Zoom so we could see our grandchildren and keep in touch with our family. Anna suggested we organise a kind of Desert Island Discs. For the non-British readers, this is a very popular and long-running radio programme, whereby a famous person is introduced and

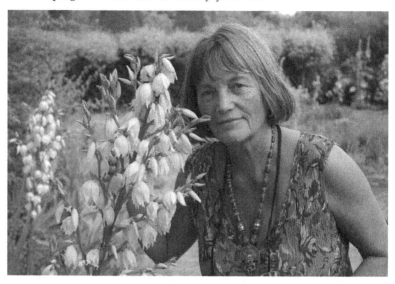

Figure 6.1 Barbara in Lutyens at a TCF meeting in 2012 aged 70 years. I have never worn make-up – not even at my own wedding.

has to select eight records which he or she would take with them if they were stranded on a desert island. The host talks about the person's life and plays each record during the programme with the person explaining why that particular song was chosen. Our family meeting was not identical but each household, there are 5 altogether with 13 people in total, selects a song which they send during the week to Sammy, our 14-year-old grandson, who lives in Chile, South America. He and his younger brother, Max, are bilingual in Spanish and English. Sammy plays the songs on disk, one at a time during the Zoom meeting. Before he plays the song, someone from the household that sent it in, explains why they chose the song and why it is important to them. One week, I chose 'You are my sunshine' because my father sang this to me when I was a little girl and I sang it to my children, my grandchildren and my great granddaughter. Sarah would have loved these family meetings.

As we could not have our special memorial dinner on the twentieth anniversary, we each sent in a song to remind us of Sarah or a song she particularly liked. Of course, Mick and I sent in Bob Dylan's 'Forever Young' as we feel that this is Sarah's song. We played it when we had the service by the River Cotahuasi where she died and we played it at her memorial service in Bury St Edmunds. If I do cry over Sarah's death, it is usually this song that will bring on my tears.

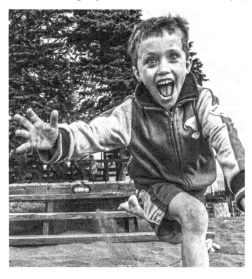

Figure 16.2 Grandson Max jumping aged 5 years.

Until two years ago, we went every year to the national gathering of TCF. We were active members helping to run some of the discussion groups, greeting the newly bereaved and first timers and helping them to settle in. Mick ran a creative writing workshop every year and also produced the TCF newsletter for several years. He often led a workshop entitled 'Grief without God' for the small number of non-believers attending. He sometimes ran and sometimes just attended a discussion group for fathers. It may seem strange in this day and age to have a father's group but it was needed partly because most of the attendees at meetings are women, partly because women seem to find it easier to express their emotions, and partly because some men find it easier to speak when women are not present. I know the men appeared to appreciate the father's group. I have said before that everyone we met at TCF had an 'at least' about their dead child such as 'At least she didn't die alone' or 'At least he made it to his brother's wedding.' In our case it was typically 'At least she wasn't murdered, raped or tortured.' It was as if each person had to appreciate that their child's death could have been worse. Mick was very moved on one occasion after a father he had met in the discussion group came to him later to talk about his dead son who had hanged himself and said 'At least he did it at home.' I have said before that everyone's loss of a child is as bad as any other person's but the *manner* of death isn't, I feel it is worse to lose a child in pain or through some despicable act of inhumanity. Ours was not like this as Sarah was full of life right through to the last moments.

The discussion group I often ran was 'Sudden death' or 'No time to say goodbye' (the same topic). The groups usually formed themselves by signing up for one of about 12 that were publicised. They usually included a group for 'Childless parents' or 'Losing your child through suicide' (or through murder) or 'What to do with your child's belongings' or 'Does grief ever end?' or 'The siblings group' and many others. No one was forced to go, there were craft activities or quiet rooms or one could go to one's bedroom and do nothing. Most people, however, went to a discussion group. The group leader checked the room early to make sure there were enough chairs, tissues and so forth. He or she checked the names of the people as they turned up and showed the people who had inadvertently arrived in the wrong room, where to go. The meeting started with the leader saying his or her name and described what had happened to their deceased child. All leaders were, of course, bereaved; we had no professionals or outsiders unless they had been invited to give the opening keynote speech.

At the meeting each person in the circle would be given the chance to say their name and how their son or daughter (or in a very few cases their sibling or grandchild) had died. This was not compulsory and if someone did not want to talk that was fine. A general discussion followed on such topics as: what had been helpful and what had been thoughtless and unfeeling. There were many tears, of course, but some laughter too and plenty of compassion. If someone cried, their neighbour would give them a hug and/or offer a tissue. The leader kept quiet as much as possible but had to make sure that one or two people did not dominate. Another task was to make sure the quiet ones wanted to be quiet and did not want to be brought in to the discussion. Some poignant and horrifying stories emerged such as the woman whose little one had drowned in the bath while being watched by a sibling and the parents who had lost all three children in a fire while they were staying at their grandmother's house.

Occasionally, I ran a discussion group called 'Losing a child abroad'. This was quite different from the 'Sudden death' group as it was more focused on practical matters. There are legal, linguistic and financial differences when one's child dies overseas compared to a death at home. The local police are meant to inform the family when this happens: this did happen for some families but it did not for ours. The insurance companies sometimes help but, again, we were told by Sarah's insurance company that it was probably a mistake and Sarah hadn't really died! The Foreign Office was useless for us and, in fact, other families felt this too. When bodies are missing in the UK, families do not have to pay for searches but we ourselves had to pay for this in Peru. The experiences of the members attending the 'losing a child abroad' group ranged from 'exceptionally good with everything happening as it should' and someone from the insurance company travelling abroad with the bereaved parent at one end of the scale, to our situation where everything that could be done in the wrong way was done that way. I remember fighting to get a death certificate, which took years to obtain. I also remember I had to get a notary public in our town to sign the Spanish translation of the details of what had happened in Peru. It took him a few seconds to sign, he charged us £50 for this signature and then he had the gall to say 'Peru, eh, that's interesting'. I was furious with him; it wasn't interesting, it was desperately sad. This group did not run every year unlike 'No time to say goodbye' and, I believe, it was less successful.

As well as discussion groups there were bigger groups such as 'the power of music' where each participant was invited to share a meaningful piece of music and say why it meant something. There was the wonderful candle lighting ceremony where we all had a lighted candle and marched in procession to leave the candle at a special place in front of the room and say our child's name. This ceremony was full of tears and we could feel the presence of all those loved ones.

Informal conversations took place too, of course. Happy and sad memories were recounted. Two of these conversation topics came up on several occasions. One was 'if you could see your dead child one more time for five minutes what would you say to him or her?' Most said something positive like 'One less day now until we meet again' but mine would be an angry conversation like 'How could you go on that dangerous white water rafting trip, Sarah, and leave your family in such turmoil?' The other conversation was a bit pointless I feel, as it asked whether it was better to lose a young child or a grown one. Well, one could make a case for and against either of these situations, but we do not get to choose, and you have to deal with what life chucks at you. We were in a minority being non-believers although TCF is for *all* religions and *no* religion. I do know though that grief at losing a child is terrible for believers and non-believers alike.

On the fortieth anniversary of the founding of TCF, Mick and I were invited to give the opening keynote address entitled 'Beacon of light and hope'. They wanted a bereaved mother and a father to speak. I had given lectures and workshops on 'Coping with bereavement: a personal perspective', Mick had not, but being a teacher, he was used to speaking. He was also used to running the creative writing workshop. In my earlier bereavement talks, I wanted to make it clear that I was not speaking as a psychologist but as a bereaved mother. Of course, at TCF I did not have to mention that I was a psychologist, I was simply one of many parents who had lost a child. The keynote talk went well I think, but as usual (at least for me) we ran out of time.

I am so much a bereaved parent now, it is so much part of my identity that we cannot really imagine how our lives would have been had Sarah not died. I was visiting Yehuda ben-Yishay, a colleague in New York, several years ago and sat in on one of his rehabilitation sessions. He asked each person in the group to write down three things about how they would describe themselves. One of my three things was that I was a bereaved mother.

For the past two years we have stopped going to the national gatherings. I think I just felt I did not need TCF now. At the beginning we needed the group very much. It gave us support, understanding and compassion. Then it was time for us to pay back and help the more newly bereaved and those suffering distress. We made some good friends there and I will always appreciate TCF but the time has come, I feel, to break our bonds.

Before continuing this chapter by once again asking Mick to contribute a story of his own, I imagine that the reader is well aware of Mick's contributions to what is in fact a tale of a marriage. I could not have completed this book without the help of Mick, and as we travelled together much of the time and as Mick was involved as a publisher of psychological tests for 13 formative years, his influence is present throughout the book. We consulted each other about each chapter. And of course we referred to my diaries that cover each day of 40 years to select what was going into the book. Occasionally, we have had to rely on Mick's own account and where this happens the text is italicised as his own. You may have noticed this in any text that concentrates on education or sport or the business of publishing – or when Mick has needed to fill in some details only available to him but is included as it explains something that has affected us both. Anyway, here is Mick's account of a ghastly incident that occurred when we were both in such a dark and painful place. Mick had to go alone to a meeting in the USA where it ended up as a disaster. He could not write or even speak about this agonising time for years but I persuaded him to explain what happened for the purposes of this book. Here is his account.

A ghastly event, as told by Mick

The year was 2000 and it was not long after Sarah had died in the white water rafting accident in Peru. For some time prior to the accident I had been committed to exhibiting some of Thames Valley Test Company's products at a conference in Washington D.C., USA. I had to go: a table had been booked, various items from stock had been delivered, some US agents were expecting me to be there; and of course I would be able to take orders from conference delegates.

The conference lasted for a couple of days and then it was time to get my flight back to England, at about 6.00 p.m. Passengers assembled at the allotted terminal expecting to be called for boarding when an announcement was made to the effect that the flight had to be delayed because of a faulty door on the plane which could not be locked shut. OK, these things happen, so maybe we'll be delayed by an hour or two until either the door is fixed or a spare one is found, or another plane can take us. I was carrying my desktop computer – quite heavy in those days twenty years ago - and a carry-on case. It was difficult to find a seat so I wandered around and eventually found floor space, holding on to computer and case not having anywhere to leave them. Several others were finding places to rest on the floor while the lucky ones who came earlier had the few seats that were around.

We waited and waited and waited as the clock got nearer to 10 o'clock. As usual there was no news from any officials and passengers were getting restless. In particular there was a bearded guy, a Brit, who was making far too much fuss, swearing a lot, extremely loud and at times shouting out obscenities about 'useless' Americans. It got so bad that I actually remonstrated with him pointing out that it hadn't been all that long ago when there had been a similar delay of a flight from Heathrow that had caused a long delay for me; it isn't just Americans that have such problems.

At last an announcement! But it was to the effect that they couldn't repair the door and that we'd all have to wait for another flight in the morning. Groans from everybody on seats and on the floor. This was going to be hell. It was, for about two more hours when past midnight another announcement was made that a number of us would be able to fly out on another flight to England in about an hour's time. We had to listen carefully as the lucky ones on the list would have their names called out. Many were called, I would think it seemed like a majority would be lucky. They formed a new queue leaving I would think about fifty of us who had not been called. Obviously we who were going to be left behind were extremely upset at being unlucky once more. I noticed the bearded guy was one of them. He was now purple with rage!

We who were left behind returned to our make shift beds on the floor and before settling down I walked to the desk to speak to the harassed officials. I was of course angry and upset, spoke too loudly to the officials, wheeled away from them into the arms of two policemen who, before I could say anything, had expertly thrown me to the floor and hand cuffed my wrists behind my back. What is going on? One of the policemen told me that I had hit him and I was going to be taken away. This was crazy. I had been carrying the heavy computer in one hand, and my carry-on case in the other. How could I hit anyone? I cried out that this was the Land of the free, some of the people on the floor were calling out for the policemen to let me go, but I was being marched away, desperately crying out for my two bags – which were picked up by one of the policemen. I felt like I was in a film.

I was taken outside and bundled into the passenger seat of a kind of van next to the driver, who was the policeman who had handcuffed me. I didn't see anyone else. He drove off and we began to converse, me stating that I certainly did not hit him and he keeping quiet. I told him, I suppose because I was hoping for some sympathy, about my need to get home because of our family bereavement at the loss of our daughter and he replied that I should be so distressed when he himself had that very morning been diagnosed with cancer of the neck as he pointed to some boil-like eruptions. I was shocked! How could he be on duty after such an experience? And how could his judgement be relied upon as being objective after that!

I was taken to what must have been a police station and shoved into a cell, the handcuffs were taken off and I was given a cup of tea. A little later a very large, policeman came in and jeeringly said I would be done for felony. I noticed the gun he had in a holster on his hip and wondered about this term 'felony' as it crept in a few times more during the night. Later I learned that the expression referred to a crime that involved violence and that heavy sentences would ensue if I was found guilty. I was scared as I knew that in America a policeman's word was sacrosanct. Deep down however my innocence held me together, it still felt like I was in a film or a dream and that reality would come back in the morning.

I hadn't long to wait in the cell before my policeman came back and took me to the van again. We drove off, this time to a prosecutor's office for me to be officially charged. The prosecutor was quiet spoken, sounded educated and listened to my story and I think he referred to a written statement by the policeman (who must have composed this while I was waiting in the cell earlier on.) Again, I felt completely gloomy as it seemed the system was built to accept a policeman's word against all comers. It was arranged that I would have to attend a court proceeding next day and that I would be picked up from a hotel at a certain time and taken to that court. The hotel was grim and breakfast in a street café was even grimmer next morning. I was in a desperately unhappy neighbourhood of lost souls with seemingly nothing to live for. I don't think I've ever felt so depressed!

At the court I didn't understand what was going on. I'd had to wait for about an hour before I was called and it was arranged that I would have to come back to the States some time in the future to face judgement in a proper court proceeding. As I left the courtroom I heard some footsteps approaching from behind quite rapidly, felt a hand on my shoulder and a pleasant looking guy smiled at me, explained that he was a defence attorney and would I like him to take on my case. I almost cried at hearing this pleasant, sympathetic voice and agreed that he should defend me. I seemed to have a friend who would genuinely listen and would perhaps believe my story! We exchanged addresses and emails and I felt for the first time that justice could evolve. I had heard about 'ambulance chasers': attorneys who chase down accident victims even before they get to hospital and how dubious the system is but this guy was the only person I could hold onto. Who else was there to fight my corner?

I made my way to the airport and was lucky enough to be able to get on to a flight to London that was leaving within the hour. On the plane I recognised some of the people who had not been able to get on the second flight last night. One of them was the bearded guy who had behaved so abominably. Being the year 2000 there were very few beards worn that year, they didn't become fashionable until about 2010 I think. Well there seemed to be only the two of us with beards.

At home and at work my lifeline turned out to be the attorney: he was caring about me, sympathetic and very sorry for our loss of Sarah. He kept in touch regularly by phone and email and told me he was working especially on my state of mind at not being able to get home at a time when our family needed to grieve together. Time dragged on for several weeks and I remained permanently anxious. Of course I discussed the issues with a number of friends, none of whom could get past their ignorance of the way justice proceeded in the USA. However, one very important point was raised by our graphic designer who stated that there must have been cameras in such a sensitive area as the boarding terminal and we should ask for them to seen as part of a properly thorough investigation. This was passed on to the attorney who still argued for a sympathetic appreciation of my state of mind at that time of night, having missed two flights and needing to get back to a grieving family. The upshot was that I sent a full coverage of Sarah's death in the white water accident that had appeared in the local newspaper: there were photos of her, the raging river in which she died, and pictures of Barbara and me mourning. It was an impressive coverage and very, very sad.

Were these final efforts going to work on the American prosecutor, who himself would, apparently, have to persuade the American police force to drop the case? A few days later I got a phone call from the attorney to say the case against me had been dropped. I could tell he was delighted and I was greatly relieved. Which argument worked on the prosecutor? The sentimental one or the properly legal one? I'll never know but I'm left with bewilderment at the mysterious ways American justice seems to work? My impression is that if the American police want to get you, they will. They are, as they say, a law unto themselves.

About a week later I got a bill for a thousand dollars from the attorney. Much later on, and to this day, I wonder whether the two policemen who got me to the ground were in fact asked to arrest the elderly bearded guy who was causing so much harm by insulting the American Nation? Was I mistakenly picked out? The two policemen could have felt they'd got their man and he was sure going to suffer. Certainly, the policemen seemed to come from nowhere. They appeared on the scene and immediately arrested me.

Mick wrote that account at a time when the whole world was still reeling from the killing of George Floyd in the USA by policemen in such an atrocious, sadistic, manner during a violent arrest. We keep thinking of all those black guys who get arrested in the USA, and here in the UK. How much worse it is for them, how they have to fight to save their lives, to escape arrest within a system where they have no means of obtaining justice, how so many of them are killed! Mick's release makes him and indeed our whole family part of racism in the sense that we, being white, can use a system to protect our innocence; we have the financial means to pay for attorneys, we can talk to witnesses; we can write letters to powerful people explaining our position, call upon witnesses, refer to newspaper articles as we did. In other words we are part of a system that is largely denied to black people and that is why black lives matter and not white lives: white lives are safe enough. We are already cared for and the world must be changed so *all* of us, white and black, are cared for; we must all have a *fair* chance to protect our innocence.

To return to TCF, I am sometimes asked to make contact with a parent, nearly always the mother, whose child has died abroad and sometimes colleagues tell me if someone they know has lost a child. In either case, I make contact and offer to speak to them or email or write. This is the kind of email I send:

Dear XX,

I hope you don't mind me contacting you but I have just heard about your (son/daughter). My eldest and beloved daughter, Sarah, died unexpectedly in a white water accident in Peru so I have some idea of the terrible time you must be going through. It is such an awful thing to outlive one's children and absolutely the wrong order. It is some years now since our loss but I remember only too well those awful days. I want to tell you that the huge waves of anguish do become less frequent and less huge over time although our lost children remain with us forever. They live in our hearts- it is not the same, of course, as having them in the flesh but they are still part of our families.

Dear Friend, I send you love, strength and compassion to get through these dreadful days and, of course, I am willing to talk to you if you feel the need. I will also understand if you want to ignore this email. Grief is exhausting, I know. Please be kind to yourself too

A hug for you and in memory of your (son/ daughter)
Barbara

So we have survived the death of a child, one of the worst experiences any parent goes through. The order is wrong, and one rages against it. We have not achieved 'closure' a word many bereaved people hate, we do not want closure, we do not want to 'get over' the death but we have become calmer and still feel an immediate bond with other bereaved parents. Sarah lives in our hearts and is still very much part of our family. Her nieces and nephews talk about her and she is a much-loved person.

17 Life today, lockdown, walks round Bury St Edmunds; Black lives matter

It is now 15 weeks since I stopped going to the gym and almost as long since the lockdown. We knew about Wuhan and the new viral infection that came to be known as Covid-19 but were not particularly worried at first. We assumed things would be OK. We were booked to go to Mallorca for a few days on 22 March. By the beginning of March 2020, Mick thought it possible we would not be able to go but, in my typically optimistic manner, I said I thought we would get there. Then on 14 March Spain locked down and stopped people travelling. The hotel where we had made a reservation said they would hold the booking until we could visit again at a future date. The airline eventually refunded the money we had paid for our flight.

On 17 March I had an email from the gym where I have been going nearly every day since February 1999. The email said that people over the age of 70 years should stop their gym membership for 12 weeks as they were at risk of catching this new virus. So I stopped my membership but the 12 weeks have long gone now and, at present there is no sign of the gym re-opening. Italy, France and Spain have all had many deaths as a result of coronavirus but the United Kingdom has had more deaths than any other European country! We locked down later than we should and our government has not behaved in a sensible or even a truthful way (Horton 2020). Trump in the USA and Bolsonaro in Brazil have behaved in an even worse fashion with terrible death rates but the UK has not come out of this well. I know at the start we believed the government, we believed lockdown should not happen too soon, we believed in developing herd immunity, but we were misled. Our son in Chile said things would get bad for the UK and, much as we hoped he would be proved wrong, he was right. Mind you, Chile has not done well either but I feel there is less protection for the poor there and the people need to be able to feed themselves so have to work or starve. It is

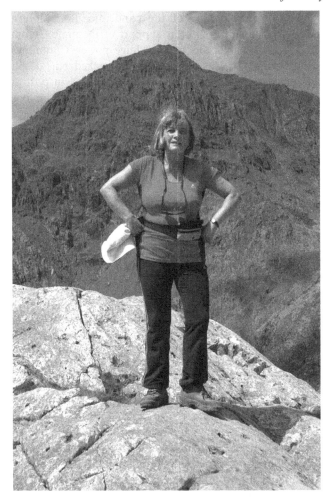

Figure 17.1 Another huge mountain conquered! It is actually Snowdon and we
descended by train.

a total disaster health and economy wise for the world. If you want to
know how the British government went so wrong I recommend Horton's
book *The Covid-19 Catastrophe: What's Gone Wrong and How to Stop
it Happening Again*. Horton is editor-in-chief of *The Lancet*, one of the
foremost medical journals, and he certainly speaks his mind on this
pandemic. Not only is he critical of our government but also of Donald
Trump of the USA and Jair Bolsonaro of Brazil too.

As well as the mishandling of the pandemic, Boris Johnson has infuriated many people through his support of Dominic Cummings, a non-elected adviser who seems to hold huge power. Cummings broke the lockdown rules and was expected to be sacked but, despite petitions and considerable media criticism, he remained in post and was strongly supported by the PM. In any other day and age, anybody with such disregard of government policy would have had to go.

Some things have improved as a result of the lock down and travel restrictions: air pollution has lessened, for example; but the pollution from plastics is almost certainly worse. Birds and animals seem bolder and one sees more of them. Many people are friendlier to one another and neighbours offer to help. As soon as lockdown was announced, we had a message from two of our neighbours offering to help in any way they could and we also had a note from the postman saying he would help with any shopping! I was quite touched by this. In fact, we have never needed help, I do a weekly shop at Waitrose where the first hour is kept for older people and those who are vulnerable. I get there about 15 minutes before opening time and stand in a queue with everyone two metres apart and hand sanitiser ready at the door of the shop.

Fortunately, we have always been allowed out for exercise. At the beginning of lockdown we were supposed to do no more than one hour's exercise a day although I have always gone out for one and a half hours each day. I know it is good for people to exercise and it also boosts the immune system. As I could not go to the gym or go swimming, I decided to walk for six miles each day and this takes me just under one and a half hours. I have not missed a day in 15 weeks, I have only repeated a walk three times and take pride in finding a different route nearly every day. Bury St Edmunds is full of footpaths, nature reserves, fields and woodlands. Within a third of a mile from our house, which is right in the middle of town, there are sheep and cattle. At the moment all the hedgerows and country lanes are full of beautiful wild flowers. Bury St Edmunds is a wonderful town full of history and historic buildings (we live in an ancient tower built into the ruins of the ancient abbey of St Edmund). I only once did less than 6 miles (five and a half miles to be precise) but regularly do more than the six miles. I also go to the local shop for a newspaper and sometimes milk after my walk so that makes another half mile.

We have had good weather on the whole, so only twice in the 15 weeks have I been caught in the rain (which I don't mind anyway, as I believe it is good for one's skin) but on two other occasions I have had to walk later in the day because the rain was so heavy. I typically go very early, leaving home between 5.30 and 6.00 a.m. I love being out and think the walks are good for my mental health. In addition to rabbits and birds, I regularly see deer, maybe a fox or a hare and once a polecat! I count the people I see on foot and there are between 6 in the 6 miles and 43 with the latter number being rare. Typically, I see between 10 and 15 people. Most are runners or walking a dog. I don't count the cyclists or the car drivers. If I go out in the afternoon though, because of morning rain, I don't count people on foot as there are too many. I always hope to manage at least one mile where I see nobody and frequently I walk for three miles with nobody around. Most people are seen in the last mile with two or three in the first mile.

Until recently, people went out at 8.00 p.m on a Thursday evening to clap for the NHS and other key workers. Mick and I went out, as did several of the others in houses along the West front. We chatted to them and felt that people seemed to be friendlier since the beginning of the pandemic. The few people I saw on my walk nearly all said 'good morning', When I go to collect the newspaper, I often see the same people and talk to them and their dogs. Near the beginning of lockdown, people also signed up to help the NHS and Francesca did this. She wasn't called on to help very often though and when she did, it was usually to deliver shopping. One thing that annoyed me was the view that anyone over the age of 70 years was vulnerable. I know most people who died of the virus were older but not all people over the age of 70 are the same. I feel fitter and healthier than many people 20 years younger than me.

The other major event that has happened during this pandemic is the rise of the Black Lives Matter movement. As Mick mentions earlier, On the 30 May 2020, George Floyd, an African-American was arrested and then killed by a white police officer with three of his colleagues standing by and not intervening. The officer kept his knee on Floyd's neck for almost nine minutes. Floyd said many times that he could not breathe and he died in these appalling circumstances. This was videoed by some of those watching and the videos were seen worldwide. We watched in horror and disbelief at the white officer who kept his knee on Floyd's neck until long after Floyd died. No doubt this has happened many times but this was the first time we had seen it. People of all races and all countries were shocked and protests were held throughout the world. Even quiet little Bury St Edmunds held a protest in support of George Floyd on Sunday 7 June. Angel Hill was filled with black, Asian and white people. Anna and Mike came and we stood (at a distance) with them. We were supposed to kneel for the length of time the officer had his knee on Floyd's neck but Mick and I could not do that, we were just too old so we stood in silence instead. Our neighbour, the dean of the cathedral, was close to us and he did kneel for the whole time. There were many speakers, all were black or Asian. One speaker started by saying he came from Brixton, which was where I grew up. I went to talk to him after his speech and he said he knew the street where I lived. We bumped elbows as we were no longer allowed to shake hands.

The officer responsible for Floyd's death was arrested for murder. His colleagues were arrested for being accessories but who knows whether or not they will be convicted. Donald Trump, the much despised president of the USA, did nothing to help the tensions in America over the Floyd incident. Instead he appeared to pour oil on the flames. The Black Lives Matter movement is still active and there are still protests in many countries. Let us hope that this will lead to a more just and fair world.

The other main difference in this pandemic period is that I have changed my work, not only using more technology but also working on Covid-19 research. This is described in the next chapter.

18 Current work and interests

I am starting this chapter on the 72nd anniversary of the National Health Service and was reminded of the 70th anniversary when I won one of the NHS parliamentary lifetime achievement awards. There were ten awards altogether for teams, services and so forth, with the one I was nominated for being considered the most prestigious. Each of five regions in the UK were requested to nominate people who had worked for 40 years in the NHS for an award. There would be five regional winners of the lifetime achievement award, each of whom would be invited to the Houses of Parliament to celebrate the 70 year anniversary and, from these, one overall winner would be chosen. Andrew Bateman, then clinical manager of the Oliver Zangwill Centre, nominated me, although the official nomination had to come from the Member of Parliament representing my constituency. This was Jo Churchill, to whom I regularly send emails protesting something or other, and, I feel, she is in the wrong party, but that is another story. I won the award for the Midlands and East region and subsequently, Mick and I went to the House of Commons in July 2018. I did not win the overall award which went to Rose Bennett, a domestic assistant from Solent NHS Trust who had worked for the NHS for 46 years. On the whole, we were pleased this award went to a domestic worker feeling that the contributions made by these workers is rarely recognised.

After the ceremony, Mick and I spent some time talking to Jo Churchill who I found myself liking even though she is in the Tory party. She arranged for her assistant, Anna Turner, to give us a tour of the Houses of Parliament. We found this interesting but were shattered by then and, after a coffee in the canteen made our goodbyes.

This is the piece that the Cambridgeshire Community Services NHS Trust wrote when it was announced I had won for the Midlands and East region:

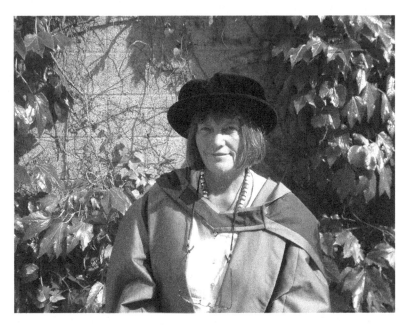

Figure 18.1 Barbara receiving an honorary doctorate from the University of East Anglia.

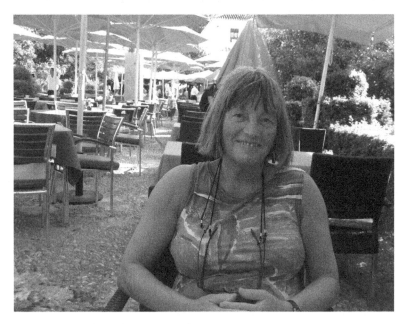

Figure 18.2 Having lunch in Marbella.

The NHS in the Midlands and East area has today (Friday 18 May) revealed that Professor Barbara Wilson OBE from Cambridgeshire Community Services NHS Trust is one of 10 it has chosen as regional champions in a prestigious competition to mark the NHS's 70th birthday.

As a resident of Bury St Edmunds, Barbara Wilson was nominated by Jo Churchill MP in the Lifetime Achievement Award category for dedicating over 40 years of her life to brain injury rehabilitation.

Barbara is esteemed for her care for patients, building bridges between practice and theory, and team work between psychologists, occupational therapists, physiotherapists and brain injured people.

She is founder of the Oliver Zangwill Centre for Neuro-psychological Rehabilitation in Ely, founder and editor of an international journal Neuropsychological Rehabilitation, author of 26 books and several instruments for testing patients, including a memory test translated into sixteen languages. She is loved by students who appreciate her devotion and encouragement.

Now retired, Professor Wilson continues to influence present and future staff in the NHS and further afield promoting the core ideas of a holistic approach to neuropsychological rehabilitation.

Professor Wilson said 'I am delighted to be shortlisted for the Lifetime Achievement Award category of the NHS70 Parliamentary Awards. Should I be successful in winning the overall award, it would be due recognition of neuropsychologists and all other professions working in brain injury rehabilitation for their essential work in assisting survivors of brain injury to lead purposeful lives.

'Being good at saving lives is admirable but we need to ensure the lives led by those saved are worthwhile and fulfilling. Such an outcome can also reduce the financial burden on statutory clinical services provided by the NHS, and lessen the stress on the lives of carers.'

Professor Wilson is representing the Midlands and East of England as they vie with other regional winners from across England for a national award to be presented at a special ceremony in the Palace of Westminster in July.

From almost 160 entries, senior experts have chosen 10 outstanding nominations, which exemplify the best of what the NHS and its partners do day in, day out.

All 10 of the champions will now be invited to the national awards ceremony, which will be held on 4 July 2018, the day before the NHS's 70th birthday. The ceremony will be hosted by

Dr Sara Kayat, NHS GP & TV Doctor best known for This Morning, Celebrity Island with Bear Grylls and GPs: Behind Closed Doors.

This was the last of five lifetime achievement awards I have won, the others being from the British Psychological Society in 2007, the International Neuropsychological Society in 2008, the National Academy of Neuropsychology in 2014, the Encephalitis Society in 2016 and the one from the NHS that I have just described.

The NHS has coped with the current pandemic but what state it will be in when this is all over, remains to be seen. At the age of 78 years, I continue to work although my work has changed over the past four months. I was going to the Oliver Zangwill Centre most Mondays until 16 March and that stopped. I hope to return at the end of August. The first time I mentioned the pandemic in my journal was on 8 March, saying the coronavirus was worrying as people were becoming infected everywhere. We did not know then if we would be able to go to Mallorca in 10 days' time or take part in any of the other travel plans I had booked for the rest of the year. I was supposed to be at a meeting in Birmingham the following week but that had been postponed. I gave a lecture at the University of East Anglia, in Norwich on 8 March (the last face-to-face talk at the time of writing). I read that the new virus may mean that all gatherings are forbidden for a while and that has proved to be true. I saw one more patient at her home near Peterborough before we were really stopped from going out and carrying on our usual life style. I also managed to continue with the gym until Tuesday 17 March. Soon after this, the Spanish government declared a state of emergency so we knew we would not be going to Mallorca in late March or to Marbella for Easter.

Instead of the gym, I walk each morning as I said in the previous chapter. The present chapter is mostly about work though and that has changed considerably. After my walk, I make sure I am up to date with emails and journal matters so that has not changed. I still do some work for my journal *Neuropsychological Rehabilitation* every single day, mostly delegating papers to an action editor but sometimes reading papers and checking details with the editorial office. I suppose I have done more writing and will say a few words about this before describing my main work interest at the moment which concerns the neuropsychological consequences of Covid-19.

The first paper I was working on during lockdown was about a patient who developed Gerstmann's Syndrome after a cardiac arrest leading to hypoxic brain damage. The syndrome is named after Josef

Gerstmann, an Austrian neuroscientist who, in 1924, described a condition with four characteristics namely an impairment in performing calculations, finger agnosia, agraphia and left-right disorientation. I saw this woman at the end of February with Heather Liddiard, a psychologist at Blackheath and, after confirming she did indeed have these four problems, and they could not be explained by other syndromes such as Balint's syndrome, apraxia or unilateral neglect, we decided to write up the case. The patient agreed to be a co-author as did the psychiatrist who had worked with the patient. We also asked Joe Mole to help and then he took over the writing up and became senior author. Joe had been a psychology assistant at the OZC before training as a clinical psychologist. He wrote a book with me and another patient (Wilson, Robertson, & Mole 2015) so I knew he had the right theoretical background and knowledge. Joe is now fully qualified and working in London. I trusted him to add the right theoretical content. The paper is almost ready to submit but we need a brain scan (the first scan was blurry and difficult to interpret). Of course, during this pandemic it is difficult to arrange for a scan so we do not know when this will happen.

I also started a paper on treating a patient with the environmental dependency syndrome. This is the man I referred to in Chapter 13 and, as I said there, this syndrome manifests itself with an array of symptoms including imitation behaviour, utilisation behaviour and inappropriate responses to cues in the environment. The paper, however, is with one of the other authors to complete and goodness knows when that will happen!

One major paper I spent a long time writing was a history of Oliver Zangwill, the man who inspired the naming of our rehabilitation centre. He is often called the father of British neuropsychology and I wanted to highlight his major contributions. I originally wrote the paper for the *History of Psychology Journal* and emailed the editor of that journal a few times. She agreed to read the draft and replied that although she thought it an interesting read, she felt it was more suited to a neuropsychology journal. This meant shortening the paper and it is now in press with *The Neuropsychologist* (Wilson in press). I write in the paper that there are a number of reasons why Zangwill is of great consequence in the history of psychology and this paper focuses on three of them. First, he is important for his views on the rehabilitation of survivors of brain damage, and in this he has had a clear although often unrecognised influence on neuropsychological rehabilitation. Second, he was responsible for making single case studies respectable and therefore acceptable in neuropsychology. Third, he made significant contributions to the understanding of problems resulting from brain damage.

While researching for the Oliver Zangwill paper, I bought a book by Shorvon and Compston (2019) on the history of Queen Square which mentioned Zangwill. I liked the book so much, I decided to read it and review it for *Neuropsychological Rehabilitation*. This is the review (reprinted with permission):

> This may seem a rather strange book to review for Neuropsychological Rehabilitation but most British neuropsychologists have been influenced one way or another by the National Hospital Queen Square (NHQS) not least because of Elizabeth Warrington and her immensely important contributions to the theoretical understanding of neuropsychological disorders. Professor Warrington actually joined the NHQS in 1953 ad was appointed professor of clinical neuropsychology in 1982. There are many characters readers will recognise throughout the book: for example, Oliver Zangwill, Tim Shallice, Alwyn Lishman, and Charles Symonds, the oft quoted man who said in 1937, 'It is not just the kind of head injury that matters but the kind of head'.
>
> The book traces the history of the NHQS since its inception in 1859 (with it being opened in 1860) until 1997. It was a voluntary hospital until 1948 when the NHS arrived but remained an independent hospital until it joined the University Hospital London NHS Trust in 1996. The work of people still alive is not referred to. Readers might be interested to know that the venerable institution came about because of two philanthropic sisters, Johanna and Louisa Chandler and their brother Edward. It began as the National Hospital for the Relief and Cure of Paralysis and Epilepsy before changing its name a few times, becoming the National Hospital for Neurology and Neurosurgery in 1990. The Institute of Neurology was established in 1950 after endless arguments, not to say opposition, to academic neurology. For example one of the neurologists at the time, Francis Walshe, despised the concept of the clinical professor!
>
> The book, although long and full of detail, is not dry. I enjoyed the mixture of politics, stories about professional individuals at the hospital, famous people treated there, constant arguments about finances, the NHS and links with the Medical Research Council, all interspersed with a chronological account of the development of the NHQS and the institute of neurology. I originally bought the book because I wanted to know what they said about Oliver Zangwill. This was because I was writing a history of Zangwill's contributions to

neuropsychology (Wilson in press) and having checked the references to him, I felt compelled to read the whole book.

Some of the professionals described are to be admired; this includes people such as Norman Dott who set up the Brain Injuries Unit near Edinburgh in the second world war. This is where Oliver Zangwill worked and where he became a neuropsychologist. I also found myself liking Roger Gilliatt who marched with CND (the campaign for nuclear disarmament) and John Marshall who invented the 'iron lung' to help those afflicted with poliomyelitis (not to be confused with the neuropsychologist of the same name who worked in Oxford).

In contrast there are people here who one would not wish to meet at all including David Ferrier who carried out some nasty animal experiments and Clifton Allbutt who made horrible comments about people in care homes that he labelled as 'imbeciles'. Even the famous Gordon Holmes seemed to be an unlikeable kind of character. Of course, they did live in different times and, perhaps should not be judged by today's standards. The authors themselves say that the British class structure began to erode in the 1960s.

There are some interesting bits of gossip and scandal. I loved the story of the hundreds of cats being looked after at the NHQS by Christine Rubin a nurse tutor who might have been a concentration camp survivor and who took the cats with her when she retired. Furthermore, she never repaid the bill for collecting all the cats! The NHQS also had to contend with scandal in the form of the deputy director of the hospital, Rosemary Aberdour, who illegally stole money by signing cheques supposedly from the chairman in order to live a lavish life style. She was eventually imprisoned.

There are a number of famous patients described including novelists Anthony Burgess, Mervyn Peake and Ian McEwan and the editor Robert McCrum. However not the cellist, Jacqueline du Pré who, I believe, was treated at the hospital by a clinical neuropsychologist, Dawn Langdon.

Other fascinating accounts are of the relationships between neurology and neurosurgery and between neurology and psychiatry. We also learn of the women appointed at the NHQS of which there were few.

In short, this is a fascinating, detailed and scholarly read. It is a beautiful book to hold and look through with plenty of photographs. I have no criticisms although some of the arguments about finances and the training of medical doctors may be of little interest to readers of this journal. I end this review with quote from page 520 of the book:

'in 2018, Queen Square remains, despite its repeated trials and tribulations, the national treasure that the Chandler siblings set out to recreate in 1859'.

In addition to writing, I have given some webinars about my work to India, Bolivia and Mexico. This meant getting used to Zoom which I had to do quickly. It is now used almost every day. I have also become involved with a World Health Organisation committee producing guidelines for brain injury rehabilitation. We have regular Webex meetings to thrash out what should go in and what is unnecessary. I have engaged in interviews about my involvement with brain injury rehabilitation and my life story via Zoom and I have listened to webinars from others. It was one of these that led to my current work in Covid-19 research which is the topic of the next chapter.

19 The neuropsychological consequences of Covid-19

On 16 May 2020 I watched a webinar on Covid-19 given by Elkhonon Goldberg from New York. I know Elkhonon, he is an interesting man who grew up in Russia and studied with Luria before moving to the USA in 1974 when he was 27 years old. I remember him telling me once that he had to pretend to be a poorly educated person in order to get a visa enabling him to leave Russia so he worked as a nursing assistant. He worked in the intensive care unit of a city hospital, mopping floors, delivering medications from the pharmacy to the unit, Every morning on arriving at 6 a.m. he had to transfer the remains of the patients who passed away during the night to the morgue (usually between five and seven people each shift). Elkhonon was given the job as a favour by an acquaintance, a physician, who was the unit chief. He was told that he didn't have to do anything, just show up, but he felt that since he took up the slot, he had to do the job, and that's what he did. The webinar was excellent. I learned there are seven coronaviruses and four are relatively mild. The three acute ones are: SARS (Severe Acute Respiratory Syndrome); MERS (Middle East Respiratory Syndrome; and the current one, SARS-Covid-2, which is the technical name for this new virus. The illness caused by SARS-COVID-2 is COVID-19.

The webinar fired my enthusiasm for getting involved in Covid-19 research. Shai Betteridge, the colleague with whom I went to Rwanda and subsequently wrote a book with (Wilson and Betteridge 2019), agreed to pay for the cost of the webinar and I agreed to write notes on this for her department. Shai explained that Jessica Fish, now working in Glasgow, was employed to work one day a week for St George's and was in charge of the research there so I should work together with Jessica. I was delighted to do this, of course, as I have always held Jessica in high regard. In this way, I became involved with researching the current pandemic. Shai arranged for me to have an honorary contract at St George's Hospital in London where she was head of department. She sent me many papers to digest and summarise. I also joined a British group of neuropsychologists working in this field and have had a number of Zoom meetings with this group.

There was another webinar on Covid-19 organised by the World Federation of Neuro-Rehabilitation (WFNR) that I also signed up to watch. This was good but very medically oriented and I thought there should have been more on neuropsychology. This became especially apparent when, after about three-quarters of the way through, a poll was conducted. Of course, I was more than happy to take part. However, I could not complete it. This is the email I wrote afterwards.

> I listened to the webinar and tried to complete the poll BUT I could not complete as there was no option for Psychologists in the professions! On the list were various doctors, OTs physical therapists, speech therapists, students and researchers but NO psychologists and no 'Other' category. I was shocked at this. Many Covid-19 survivors who have been seriously ill are likely to have need of neuropsychological help with cognitive, emotional and behavioural problems. We are working with the British Psychological Society and The Division of Neuropsychology on this ... Anyway, I thought I would flag this up.

As a result of this email, I was invited a) to produce a piece for the next WFNR newsletter and b) take part in the next webinar. I wrote a short piece for the newsletter which was as follows:

> We know that many organs can be affected by the Corona virus, Covid-19, including the lungs, heart, blood, digestive system and brain. The virus can directly affect the brain although the mechanisms by which this occurs are not clear: it could be a direct cause or a secondary effect (or both). However, because evidence of the virus has been found in the cerebral spinal fluid of patients, this suggests a direct cause (Goldberg webinar May 2020).
>
> Of those who are rendered severely ill by the virus, some will go on to develop hypoxic brain damage, encephalitis, stroke, multiple sclerosis, or epilepsy and thus may have problems that require a referral to a neuropsychologist. Some 6% of Covid-19 patients admitted to hospital are likely to develop encephalitis; strokes are not infrequent, and these can be both ischaemic and haemorrhagic. In the United Kingdom, haemorrhagic strokes are seen in patients in their 50s to 80s while in the United States of America, ischaemic strokes are reported in younger people in their 30s and 40s (ibid.).

Indeed, Covid-19 may even present as stroke as reported in four patients in the USA (Avula et al in press).

In another webinar presented by WFNR, Feng observed that one in four people admitted to hospital have CNS involvement but only 3% had stroke; and that COVID-19 can cause sudden strokes in young people with no risk factors. One interesting point was his claim that ALL Covid-19 strokes died in hospital, while only 10% of other stroke patients died there! In general, there is a higher mortality rate if Covid-19 patients are admitted to hospital with neurological symptoms. Ellul et al (2020), looking at 153 people seen in British hospitals, found that cerebrovascular events predominated in older patients. Conversely, altered mental status, while present in all ages, had a disproportionate representation in the young.

Those who have spent a long time in intensive care may be left with lasting cognitive impairment. This is not to mention the possibility of long term emotional consequences such as anxiety, stress, depression and insomnia, All these problems are typically assessed and treated by neuropsychologists. Of the cognitive problems, memory, attention, executive deficits, verbal fluency, slowed information processing and speech and language problems have all been reported (Ritchie, Chan and Watermeyer 2020). An Indian colleague, Jwala Narayanan, has also reported a 62 year old patient who developed Covid-19, then had a stroke and was left with Balint's syndrome (Narayanan, Evans and Wilson 2020). This syndrome is rare and is comprised of three components: namely, psychic paralysis of gaze or optic apraxia, which is an inability to look voluntarily into the peripheral field; optic ataxia, which is an inability to localise in space or manually point to visually presented objects; and simultanagnosia where, despite adequate visual acuity, it is impossible to process more than one visually presented object at a time.

All of the above reports and observations suggest that many survivors of Covid-19 are likely to require neuropsychological rehabilitation which, at present, is severely underfunded.

I mention in the article for WFNR that an Indian colleague, Jwala Narayanan, identified a patient with Balint's syndrome after being diagnosed with Covid-19 and then developed a stroke. Jwala emailed me about this patient on 10 June 2020 and I said as this was probably the first Covid-19 patient to be identified with this rare syndrome, we should write her up. Jon Evans, currently active in the International Neuropsychological Society (INS), had recently said the INS were looking for interesting Covid-19 patients so Jwala, Jon and I worked together and now the paper has been accepted. We said the main messages were first that a rare syndrome might sometimes follow a stroke caused by Covid-19 and second, that neuropsychologists should be aware of this when assessing patients with a diagnosis of Covid-19 as the syndrome is easy to miss and often mistaken for blindness. As more patients diagnosed with Covid-19 are likely to be referred for a neuropsychological assessment and treatment, and some of these will have had stroke or hypoxic brain damage, we need to ensure that such rare syndromes are not overlooked.

In the past, I have given master classes for Jason Shelley, his wife Helen Edwards and their company ABI Solutions. These were stopped or postponed during the lock down period but I suggested to Jason that I could do a webinar on the neuropsychological consequences of Covid-19. He agreed to this and I filmed a talk for him in July 2020. I am also going to give a talk on the topic at St George's Hospital in August 2020, if lock down is not reintroduced because of a second wave of the coronavirus.

All this work began because Shai Betteridge and St George's Hospital wanted me to carry out an audit of the patients referred to the neuropsychology department and, for this, I am grateful. Jessica Fish and I have regular telephone discussions about the audit. We are conducting these in an attempt to characterise the neuro-psychological needs of the people with Covid-19 seen within the department. The specific questions are 'What are the reasons for referral of patients with COVID to neuropsychology? What, if any, cognitive, emotional and behavioural difficulties are they experiencing? What is the functional impact of these difficulties?' As we do not know the long-term consequences of these problems, we need to find out if they persist or resolve over time.

We are also interested in discovering whether there are differences between those who had an underlying condition when they developed Covid-19 and those who did not, in terms of demographics, cognition, behaviour and emotional well-being. Through this audit we hope to be able to better understand the needs of this patient group, to inform the service we provide for them, and to share this knowledge with colleagues.

I have started to analyse the St George's data and, like other reports in the UK, we are finding a predominance of ethnic minority groups in those referred, typically they have been in intensive care, with most referrals being for cognitive and mood problems. The cognitive problems are typically memory, executive difficulties and slow information processing. Some emotional problems such as flatness of affect have been noted but only one behaviour problem to date. In addition to the hospital audit, we are collaborating with several countries around the world to see if their referrals to neuropsychology, are similar to those seen at St George's Hospital. So far, Caterina Pistarini from Italy is the most engaged internationally and her group have just sent in some preliminary results.

20 Final thoughts

Music, art and literature have played their part in my life at varying levels, as they do of course in many people's lives. I am, or have been at times, a member of the National Gallery, The British Museum, and the Royal Academy, and have attended many national exhibitions but I wouldn't say my interest for any specific artist or historical period or particular medium is particularly profound. I am much more of a scientist I suppose and am absorbed by medical and mental aspects of illness and recovery. It would be true to say that Mick is probably more interested in the art world than I am. He certainly looks forward more than I do to visiting exhibitions and gets absorbed in observing artefacts and paintings. As far as literature is concerned, I am an obsessive reader of all kinds of books and I'm never without a book or two to read each week while Mick, as an ex-teacher of English, has maintained an interest in novels, poetry and plays. We both love our trips to the theatre to see Shakespeare's plays and have been at times members of the Royal Shakespeare Company at Stratford-upon-Avon. Again, I would say that Mick's interest in Shakespeare is far greater than mine although I do love going to the theatre. As far as music is concerned, apart from Mick's deep interest in jazz neither of us has been a follower of any specific genre. We are not collectors of disks for example and apart from one particular stage in our married life, have never had a gramophone or record player for lengthy listening of music. Of course we both have our favourite records, pieces of music and songs just as anybody does and we wouldn't have difficulty in naming our desert island choices. The one exception is our love of Bob Dylan's songs, which we have collected throughout our married life, ever since we first heard him in the early 1960s when living in Colchester. As for films, since moving to the centre of Bury St. Edmunds six years ago and living within five minutes' walk of an excellent Arts Cinema, which has its own restaurant, we have both become ardent film buffs and love our visits to the cinema to see the latest films. We'd be lost without our cinema and it's such a privilege for us to be an elderly couple walking hand in hand to the cinema, having a nice meal, and then watching a good film, and maybe a glass of wine and a chat afterwards.

The pandemic has brought me more work and of a different kind, although of course I would rather it had not occurred as it has been so devastating. We would not have believed this time last year that such a thing could cause so much havoc in such a short space of time. Mick and I would love to have access to an antibody test as I said earlier, we feel we may well have had the virus in February 2020. If a reliable antibody test is made available, however, we will not, at our age, be top of the priority list! In the meantime I have been able to get on with this book because of the accompanying lockdown for the last 16 weeks. For that I am grateful and will have to hope the reader feels the same way!

Our daily life is of course limited by the lockdown, which in itself is not too bad for us: I am able to get on with most of my work at home, consisting of research on the internet and the writing of papers plus many discussions with colleagues via Zoom or Webex regarding the shape and nature of work in the future and ways of reacting to the effects of the pandemic particularly when brain injury is involved. I don't have to worry about the house or garden although I am responsible for 90 per cent of the cooking – which I find enjoyable as it is such a change from work. Mick, in his retirement, looks after the house and garden and is always around to dot the i's and cross the t's of any writing I may do. In effect, as an ex-teacher of English, he is a remarkably good editor of my work, and saves me a lot of time not needing to consult with professional editors or proofreaders. And I always have my diaries dating back to 1979 to consult when I am considering what to include in the autobiography.

Well that was going to be about it. I was going to finish the whole autobiography with some kind of comforting sentence to bring it to a satisfactory ending – until something happened just now which forces me to an unforeseen conclusion illustrative of the kind of interruption that makes the life of a clinical neuropsychologist so interesting. An accurate reflection of the way we work!

So, today we had our mini conference of the Neuropsychological Rehabilitation Special Interest Group by Zoom. This is the annual two-day meeting that should have been in Vienna. Being chair of the group, I always give the opening talk. I try to make this challenging, controversial or unusual. This year, my talk was entitled 'Similarities and differences between bereaved parents and parents of someone with a very severe brain injury: what can we do to help?' I gave the talk which I think was well received, I had many emails from people saying how much they had appreciated it. Then one email came in from a mother, a psychologist, whose son had been brain injured. It was a really sad email and I found myself in tears over the story. I replied and said I hoped that when this pandemic was over, we should meet, not as psychologists but as mothers who had endured what mothers should not have to endure.

I wrote an editorial in my journal on this topic and have chosen to end this autobiography today with this same editorial as in some ways the words summarise my position and the way I'm feeling at this time of my life.

'Similarities and differences between bereaved parents and parents of a person with a very severe brain injury: What can we do to help?

As a clinical neuropsychologist, I work with people who have sustained a brain injury and their families. Some of these patients will have sustained a very severe injury and remain in a prolonged disorder of consciousness (PDOC). I also happen to be a bereaved parent: my oldest child, Sarah, died in a white water rafting accident in Peru in May 2000 at the age of 36 years (Wilson 2020a). Consequently, I often feel a close connection with the families of patients who have sustained a brain injury, particularly those in a PDOC, and this has led me to reflect upon how the two groups might be similar and how they might differ.

Ostensibly, there are similarities and differences faced by parents whose loved one has died and parents whose loved one has survived a very severe brain injury. Both have lost the person they once knew, both grieve, may be filled with regret and/or guilt, face levels of stress and changes in well being, and both are likely to obtain support from others in the same situation. The main difference is that families of a very severely brain injured person face an ambiguous loss: theirs is a daily loss without an immediate end. Their loved one is alive and has a sleep/wake cycle, moves, makes noises and reacts to stimuli. Despite this, the loved one does not initiate communication or social interaction and may appear unreactive to anything meaningful. The brain injured person may also appear to be in pain or distress and show signs of sadness, even at times shedding tears. Experiencing no interaction, communication or behaviour challenges our understanding of people, and as, some report, 'life itself'. Family members in these circumstances cannot grieve their loss fully; they may constantly be searching for answers and this complicates and delays the process of mourning, sometimes resulting in unresolved anguish.

While formal and certainly more abundant assistance and support is available to bereaved parents through organisations such as The Compassionate Friends, and the Encephalitis Society (which supports families who have lost someone because of encephalitis), there do not appear to be similar organisations for severely brain damaged people – apart from an online support group run by Celia and Jenny Kitzinger, and of course the work of clinical psychologists and neuropsychologists, professionally available to both groups initially.

My colleague, Anita Rose, who is also a clinical neuropsychologist, indicated that one-third of the caregivers of people with a severe traumatic brain injury have clinically significant symptoms of mood disorders such as depression and anxiety and they can sometimes be described as suffering 'prolonged grief disorder'. Family members show high levels of loss and distress, both physical and emotional changes in well being, high levels of carer burden and lowered levels of coping. Dr Rose goes on to say that support for these families involves good communication and the provision of information about the clinical state of the patient, the prognosis, available treatments, the treatment plan and any necessary investigations. This is in addition to practical and emotional support. Should the family have questions, names of appropriate team members should be provided and information as to how to access these team members supplied. Families should also be involved in goal setting and care planning and they should be informed of the evaluation of progress; they should be involved in joint assessments where appropriate; and be involved in decisions made in the patient's best interests. After all, families know the patients better than the staff looking after them. Information fact sheets and booklets should be made available as well as signposts to services and how to meet other families in a similar situation if this is considered desirable. Other practical support may include assistance with managing finances, helping with housing and care homes and transport. The psychologist should always have available, paper handkerchiefs, a cup of tea and a listening ear.

Family support may be facilitated by staff or experienced family members who can create informal opportunities to build contacts, arrange family meetings, guide access to peer support either face to face or via online resources. Families can be shown how to engage in therapy for the patient: for example, teaching them how to give a gentle massage or stretching exercises; conducting basic daily care tasks; and providing stimulation. Families may also need to be shown how to take respite and have the confidence to leave their loved one when they need a break or need to go home.

Psychologists can, of course, offer counselling and support although family members may not be ready for this in the early stages. This is also true of bereaved parents, who may not be ready to accept help early on; so for both groups the offer of support should be repeated after an interval. Counselling to families of people in a PDOC should be provided by professionals with understanding of the condition so that facts not fiction are provided.

While these kinds of support from professionals are important, many of them can be continued and extended within self-help groups for the bereaved. This, then, may be another difference. Those with a severe brain injury still require professional care whereas the dead person obviously has no need of this. I suggest, however, that both groups, are changed by the experience. TCF is a club whose members seem to have, despite the most awful losses, grown as human beings, exhibiting dignity and exceptional empathy to others faced with the same agonising loss. This may well be true for the families of those with a very severe brain injury if they are given similar opportunities to meet together.

It is not only very severe brain injury that changes outlook on life: Richard Houghton (2018) in a book about sudden cardiac arrest (SCA) and, himself a survivor with very mild, if any, brain injury, says 'I also gained some things that I wouldn't have done apart from the SCA. I have learned humility for those less fortunate than me and gained greater compassion' (P61). It is worth noting that this term, compassion, refers to empathy and feeling with others and is not pity: it is regarded as the highest of the virtues in all major religious traditions.

As a bereaved parent I needed certain things soon after my daughter died and I am not sure whether these needs are similar or different for other families. I needed to read what other bereaved parents felt and thought. It was important to learn from others with the same experience. I needed to know there were good people in the world and that it was possible to lead a meaningful life after losing a child.

In summary, as a bereaved parent, I learned the following things:

Grief isn't one constant feeling. It comes in huge waves that wash over one.

The waves decrease in frequency over time but can still be as overwhelming as ever.

It is still possible to have moments where one can smile, feel hungry, do 'normal' things even early on.

Grief is exhausting and it slows one's cognitive functioning.

There is an immediate bond with other bereaved parents (it crosses all barriers).

A great gift, early on is to let us talk and let us cry.

Don't say 'I don't know what to say' – if you know the deceased person tell some anecdote (I remember when…). If you don't know the person say "tell me about (XX) what was s/he like?

Don't say 'I couldn't live with it'. We HAVE to live with it – there is no choice.

Don't say 'Have you achieved closure?' This is one of the expressions most hated by bereaved parents because they don't want to forget.

If you can't speak, a gentle touch may suffice to show your compassion.

One worries less about unimportant things. Our priorities change.

Most people were good – some didn't cope.

Some people one didn't expect much from came up trumps.

Someone said to us early on 'Your address book will change' and it has.

Good and bad things in the early days are remembered with heightened awareness.

Letting us come to terms in our own way and at our own speed is important.

We are all part of a terrible yet special club that no one wants to be in but we need each other.

When we are with others in the same situation, we don't have to hide our feelings; we don't have to wonder 'do they know'. Everyone's in a similar boat.

One final area where I do not know if this is a similarity or a difference is that all bereaved parents have an 'at least'.

'At least she didn't die in agony.'

'At least he died at home.'

'At least he saw his brother's wedding.'

'At least we had a body to bury.'

One has to deal with the hand that has been dealt and this is true of both groups.

I end with a quote by Haruki Murakami from the 2018 Cardiac Arrest book as this seems to sum up the plight of all families facing a huge life changing event.

'And once the storm is over, you won't remember how you made it through, how you managed to survive. You won't even be sure, whether the storm is really over. But one thing is certain. When you come out of the storm, you won't be the same person who walked in. That's what this storm's all about.'

References

Allen, R.E., Fowler, H.W., & Fowler, F.G. (1990). *The concise Oxford dictionary of current English*. Oxford: Oxford University Press.

Arango Lasprilla, J.C., Wilson B.A., & Olabarrieta Lancia, L. (Eds) (2020). *Principios de rehabilitacion neuropsychologica*. Mexico City: Manuel Moderno.

Archibald, S.J., Kerns, K.A., Mateer, C.A., & Ismay, L. (2005). Evidence of utilization behavior in children with ADHD. *Journal of the International Neuropsychological Society*, 11(4), 367–375.

Avula, A., Nalleballe, K., Narula, N., Sapozhnikov, S., Dandu, V., Toom, S., Glaser, A., & Elsayegh, D. (in press). COVID-19 presenting as stroke. *Brain, Behaviour and Immunity*.

Chadwick, H. (2020). The Magdalena Project in memory of Venice Manley (downloaded 22 May). https://themagdalenaproject.org/

Ellul, M., Benjamin, L., Singh, B., Lant, S., Michael, B.D., Easton, A., Kneen, R., Defres, S., Sejvar, J., & Solomon, T. (in press). Neurological associations of COVID-19. *The Lancet Neurology*.

Feng, W. (2020,May). The impact of COVID-19 on neurorehabiltative care & research (webinar by the World Federation of NeuroRehabilitation).

Geschwind, N. (1965). Disconnexion syndromes in animals and man. II. *Brain*, 88(3), 585–644. doi:10.1093/brain/88.3.585

Ghosh, A., & Dutt, A. (2010). Utilisation behaviour in frontotemporal dementia. *Journal of Neurology, Neurosurgery & Psychiatry*, 81(2), 154–156.

Goldberg, E. (2020, May). Covid-19 and the brain (webinar, organised by the Luria Neuroscience Institute, New York).

Harmer, M. (1982). *The forgotten hospital*. London: Springwood Books.

Horton, R. (2020). *The Covid-19 catastrophe: What's gone wrong and how to stop it happening again*. Cambridge: Polity books.

Ishihara, K., Nishino, H., Maki, T., Kawamura, M., & Murayama, S. (2002). Utilization behavior as a white matter disconnection syndrome. *Cortex*, 38 (3), 379–387.

Lagarde, J., Valabrègue, R., Corvol, J.C., Le Ber, I., Colliot, O., Vidailhet, M., & Levy, R. (2013). The clinical and anatomical heterogeneity of environmental dependency phenomena. *Journal of Neurology*, 260(9), 2262–2270.

Lefanu, S. (2014). Marjorie Blandy 1887–1937. In C. Tomalin, J. Ashworth, M. Drabble, S. Lefanu, E. Feinstein, & S. Limb (Eds), *Breaking bounds: Six Newnham lives* (pp. 53–65). Cambridge: Newnham College.

Lhermitte, F. (1983). 'Utilization behaviour'and its relation to lesions of the frontal lobes. *Brain*, 106(2), 237–255.

Lhermitte, F. (1986). Human autonomy and the frontal lobes. Part II: Patient behavior in complex and social situations: The 'Environmental Dependency Syndrome'. *Annals of Neurology*, 19, 335–343.

Lhermitte, F., Pillon, B., & Serdaru, M. (1986). Human autonomy and the frontal lobes. Part I. *Annals of Neurology*, 19, 326–334.

Loschiavo-Alvares, F., Fish, J., & Wilson, B.A. (2018). Applying the comprehensive model of neuropsychological rehabilitation to people with psychiatric conditions. *Clinical Neuropsychiatry*, 15, 83–93.

Loschiavo-Alvares, F., & Wilson, B.A. (Eds) (2020). *Neuropsychological rehabilitation for psychiatric diseases*. Guaraja: Artesa.

Macniven, J.A., Poz, R., Bainbridge, K., Gracey, F., & Wilson, B.A. (2003). Case study: Emotional adjustment following cognitive recovery from 'persistent vegetative state': Psychological and personal perspectives. *Brain Injury*, 17(6), 525–533.

Marin, R.S., & Gorovoy, I.R. (2014). Echothymia: Environmental dependency in the affective domain. *J Neuropsychiatry Clin Neurosci*, 26(1), 92–96.

Menon, D.K., Owen, A.M., Williams, E.J., Minhas, P.S., Allen, C.M.C., Boniface, S.J., & Pickard, J.D. (1998). Cortical processing in persistent vegetative state. *Lancet*, 352(9123), 200.

Narayanan, J., Evans, J., & Wilson, B.A. (2020). Balint's syndrome as a post-COVID 19 complication: A case from southern India. *INS*, 3, 27–30.

Owen, A.M., Coleman, M.R., Boly, M., Davis, M.H., Laureys, S., & Pickard, J.D. (2006). Detecting awareness in the vegetative state. *Science*, 313, 1402.

Proceedings of the Association of British Neurologists, University of Oxford, 3 April – 5 April 2002 (2002). *J. Neurol. Neurosurg. Psychiatry*, 73, 213–236. doi:10.1136/jnnp.73.2.213

Ritchie, K., Chan, D., & Watermeyer, T. (2020). The cognitive consequences of the COVID-19 epidemic: Collateral damage?. *Brain Communications*. http s://doi.org/10.1093/braincomms/fcaa069

Roberts, B., Rose, A., Wilson, B.A., Fish, J., & Florschutz, G. (2018). Treating environmental dependency syndrome in a person with an acquired brain injury: An ABAB design. Poster presented at a meeting of The Special Interest Group in Neuropsychological Rehabilitation, Cape Town, South Africa. (See INS website).

Schnakers, C., Majerus, S., Goldman, S., Boly, M., Van Eeckhout, P., Gay, S., Pellas, F., Bartsch, V., Peigneux, P., Moonen, G., et al. (2008). Cognitive function in the locked-in syndrome. *Journal of Neurology*, 255(3), 323–330.

Shorvon, S., & Compston, A., with contributions from A. Lees, M.Clark, & M. Rossor (2019). *Queen Square: A history of the National Hospital and its Institute of Neurology*. Cambridge: Cambridge University Press.

Solms, M. (1995). Is the brain more real than the mind?. *Psychoanalytic Psychotherapy*, 9(2), 107–120.

Swindell, P. (Ed.) (2018). *Life after cardiac arrest*. Braintree: Sudden Cardiac Arrest UK.

Tomalin, C., Ashworth, J., Drabble, M., Lefanu, S., Feinstein, E., & Limb, S. (2014). *Breaking bounds: Six Newnham lives*. Cambridge: Newnham College.

Warlow, C. (2002). ABN medal award 2002. *Journal of Neurology, Neurosurgery and Psychiatry*, 73(2), 213.

Wilson, B.A. (2002). Towards a comprehensive model of cognitive rehabilitation. *Neuropsychological Rehabilitation*, 12, 97–110.

Wilson, B.A. (2019). How long might recoveries continue after very severe brain injury?. *Journal of Clinical Review and Case Reports*, 4(2), 1–3.

Wilson, B.A. (2020a). *The story of a clinical neuropsychologist*. Abingdon: Routledge.

Wilson, B.A. (2020b). Editorial: Similarities and differences between bereaved parents and parents of a person with a very severe brain injury: What can we do to help?. *Neuropsychological Rehabilitation*, 30(2), 163–165.

Wilson, B.A. (2020c). Obituary for Don Stuss. *The Neuropsychologist*, 9, 11.

Wilson, B.A. (2020d). Oliver Zangwill (1913-1987): The father of British neuropsychology. *The Neuropsychologist*, 10, 65–72.

Wilson, B.A., & Bainbridge, K. (2014). Kate's story: Recovery takes time so don't give up. In B.A. Wilson, J. Winegardner, & F. Ashworth (Eds), *Life after brain injury: Survivors' stories* (pp. 50–62). Hove: Psychology Press.

Wilson, B.A., & Betteridge, S. (2019). *Essentials of neuropsychological rehabilitation*. New York: Guilford Press.

Wilson, B.A., & Okines, T. (2014). Quality of life with locked-in syndrome. In B.A. Wilson, J. Winegardner, & F. Ashworth (Eds), *Life after brain injury: Survivors' stories* (pp. 75–83). Hove: Psychology Press.

Wilson, B.A., & Wilson, M.J. (2004). *First year: Worst year: Coping with the unexpected death of our grown up daughter*. Chichester: John Wiley & Sons.

Epilogue

Since completing this book and while checking details on 11 July 2020, few things have happened. The lockdown is slowly beginning to ease and we are taking my sister-in-law, Carol, to a restaurant today for a delayed birthday meal. From 4 July 2020 we were allowed to have people from one other household in the house so we had our daughter, Anna and her husband Mike, for dinner. Anna also brought great granddaughter, Amélie, round on 6 July. We have met her in our garden and in the park during lockdown but not inside our house. So things are slowly getting back to some sort of normality although we are fearful of another surge of the pandemic. The gyms are not open yet so I am still walking six miles each day (I have not missed a single day yet) and in 116 days I have only repeated a walk on three occasions. I keep finding new paths to explore.

In December 2020 effective vaccines against the virus started to be administered to various populations throughout the world.

Printed in the United States
by Baker & Taylor Publisher Services